DR. ROGER GARCIA

Foreword by Pamela W. Smith, M.D., MPH
Best-Selling Author & International Speaker

AGED *to* PERFECTION

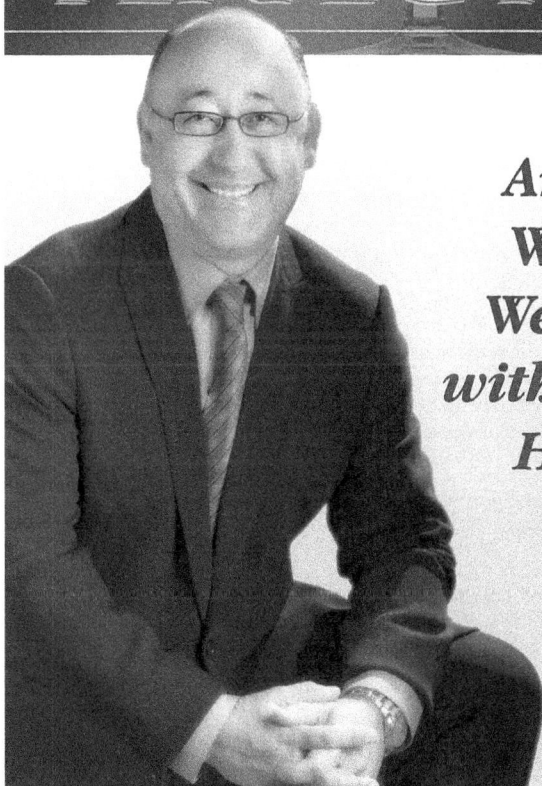

Anti-aging, Wellness & Weight Loss with Natural Hormones

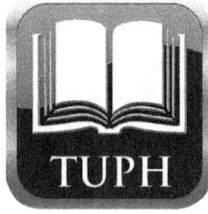

THE ULTIMATE PUBLISHING HOUSE (TUPH)

US HEADQUARTERS

The Ultimate Publishing House (TUPH)

P.O. Box 1204

Cypress, Texas, U.S.A. 77410

49540 – 80 GLEN SHIELDS AVENUE, TORONTO, ONTARIO
CANADA, L4K 2B0
Telephone: 647.883.1758 Fax: 416-228-2598

www.ultimatepublishinghouse.com and www.agedtoperfectionbook.com

E-mail: info@ultimatepublishinghouse.com

US OFFICE: Ordering Information

Quantity Sales: COMPANIES, ORGANIZATIONS, INSTITUTIONS,
AND INDUSTRY PUBLICATIONS.

Quantity discounts are available on bulk purchases of this book for reselling, educational purposes, subscription incentives, gifts, sponsorship, or fundraising. Unique books or book excerpts can also be fashioned to suit specific needs such as private labelling with your logo on the cover and a message from or a message printed on the second page of the book. For more information please contact our Special Sales Department at The Ultimate Publishing House.

Orders for college textbook or course adoption use.
Please contact the Ultimate Publishing House

Tel: 647 883 1758

TUPH is a registered trademark of The Ultimate Publishing House

Printed in Canada.

Aged to Perfection, by Dr. Roger Garcia

ISBN: 978-0-9819398-6-5

DISCLAIMER

The information and advice contained within this book is based on the research and the personal and professional experiences of the author. The reader should seek the advice of a trusted health care professional regarding the risks, benefits, indications, and contra-indications of all suggestions, preparations, or procedures discussed in this book. The publisher and author are not responsible for any adverse effects or consequences, directly or indirectly, resulting from the information contained within this book.

Dedication

For my girls,
James, Jaymes, and Stone

Acknowledgments

Gratitude is a powerful emotion that conveys understanding, humility, and love. I found myself deep in this emotion while writing this book and upon reflection of how many people had to come into my life to make it happen. These newfound friendships and this experience has forever changed and blessed me. God sure does work in mysterious ways.

To my wife, Jamie, who always picks me up when I am down and knows when to let me fall when I need it. This book simply would not have been possible without your patience and encouragement. Thank you for not allowing the household to disintegrate during the writing of this book.

To my twin girls, Jaymes and Stone, age 6. The world cannot hold the love I have for you. The most difficult part of having to work, including writing this book, is the lost time spent away from you. You are true blessings in my life and I will always hold you in my heart and in my prayers.

To my mother and father, whose sacrifices and encouragement allowed me to live my dreams and showed me through their example, that a little faith really can move mountains.

To my brothers, George and David, and my sister, Emma, though we may never agree on all things, in the things that matter, love of family and God, we travel the same path.

To Roger and Karen Boger, who awoke me from my malaise and made me realize my potential.

To Felicia Pizzonia, who strongly believed in this project from the beginning and gave me the name of this book. For all your talents as a publisher, you shine more brightly as a trusted advisor and friend.

To Dr. Paul Savage, who helped me see when I was blind and guided me down the path of understanding of real health and wellness.

To Dr. Ron Rothenberg, who showed me what it means to feel and act "ageless."

To Dr. David West, for your friendship and your gracious participation in writing a section of this book.

To Dr. Pamela Smith, for writing the Foreword of this book despite the many demands placed upon you by your teaching and lecture schedule. I am grateful for the training I received from the fellowship program as it helped me to see wellness from greater heights of clarity.

To Kendall Cho, whose life story is a constant inspiration to me and for helping me to realize that all things are possible.

To Richard Emmanuel, whose personality and encouragement made me feel like a shining star on Broadway.

To my friends and colleagues at BodyLogicMD, who gave me strength and knowledge through selflessly giving of your time and expertise. I will be forever grateful and I am proud to call you my brethren.

To the many physicians and mentors, named and unnamed, who guided me through the uncharted waters called integrative medicine. Special thanks to Dr. Mark Gordon, Dr. Sangeeta Pati, Dr. Pam Smith, and Dr. Jonathan Wright.

To my friends and colleagues at the Bellevue Hospital in Bellevue, Ohio, who always encouraged me in this endeavor in their own special way. Our shared experiences in the ED have forged a special bond that can never be broken.

To my friends and colleagues at North Central Emergency Services, thank you for the friendship that only comrades in arms can understand.

To my staff, Michele Alban, Tracey Holcomb, and Lee Mayle, who work countless hours in the office and on the phone to ensure a great patient experience and keep the office running smoothly. You are the true heroes of the office.

To the many physicians and personalities who have contributed to the advancement of integrative medicine and the use of bioidentical hormones. Through their efforts, many have come to healing. To name them all is impossible but special thanks to Dr. Jeffrey Bland, Dr. John Lee, Dr. Edward Lichten, Dr. Sheri Lieberman, Ms. Robin McGraw, Dr. Joseph Mercola, Dr. Abraham Morgentaler, Dr. Christiane Northrup, Dr. Mehmet Oz, Dr. Perricone, Dr. Diana Schwarzbein, Dr. Norman Shealy, Ms. Suzanne Somers, Dr. Andrew Weil, Dr. Julian Whitaker, and Ms. Oprah Winfrey.

Last but not least, to my patients, who have shared their private trials and tribulations with me. I am truly humbled and privileged to be able to help and participate in your path toward healing if only in some small way.

A Short History of Medicine

2000 B.C. - *"Here, eat this root."*
1000 B.C. - *"That root is heathen, say this prayer."*
1850 A.D. - *"That prayer is superstition, drink this potion."*
1940 A.D. - *"That potion is snake oil, swallow this pill."*
1985 A.D. - *"That pill is ineffective, take this antibiotic."*
2000 A.D. - *"That antibiotic is artificial. Here, eat this root."*

~Author Unknown

FOREWORD

by Pamela W. Smith, M.D., MPH

There is a sea change occurring in the way medicine will be practiced in the future. This change will not be borne of any new profound discovery in pharmacology or by any innovative diagnostic medical device. Nor will this change be the result of any policy shift emerging from the legislative halls of government. The source of this paradigm shift in medicine may come as a bit of a surprise to you. Happily, it is coming from the physicians themselves. More and more practitioners like Dr. Garcia are leading the way in re-establishing the art of the practice of medicine. Dr. Garcia, in his altruistic calling to help people be as healthy as they can possibly be and enhance their quality of life for as long as they live, is spearheading a new field of medicine called Metabolic and Anti-Aging Medicine.

Doctors are uniting together in recognizing that treating symptoms alone is not only unfulfilling for them professionally, but also failing the patient in aiding their return to optimal health. There has emerged among the more enlightened doctors the realization that no two people are alike and that individualized care is called for. Recognizing our bio-individuality and the role that "body-mind-spirit" plays in Metabolic Medicine is key. Dr. Garcia is correct; it is not about being obsessed with youth. It is about immersing oneself into a healthful and proactive process of aging whereby confidence, competence, vision, memory, and mobility are maintained until the very end of life.

If you are truly motivated and willing to initiate the necessary changes in your lifestyle and dietary habits as well as addressing the relationships and spiritual issues in your life, then aging well may very well be in your future.

These new types of practitioners, like Dr. Garcia, have been astute enough to seek specialized training through a two-year fellowship/masters degree program offered by the University of South Florida College of Medicine. Please seek out these practitioners. Your hormones and nutritional status are responsible for countless metabolic processes throughout your body and are all linked in a confoundingly complex web of interaction. It takes a fellowship-trained metabolic specialist to sort out exactly what you, individually, require for optimal health to occur. Read this book, see a doctor like Dr. Garcia, and prepare to make meaningful changes to aid you in enjoying optimal health for the remainder of your life.

In good health,

Pamela W. Smith, M.D., MPH
Co-Director, Masters Program in Medical Sciences with a Concentration in Metabolic and Nutritional Medicine, University of South Florida College of Medicine

TABLE OF CONTENTS

Introduction

"The superior doctor prevents sickness. The mediocre doctor attends to impending sickness. The inferior doctor treats actual sickness."

Ancient Chinese proverb

I believe that we are meant to enjoy the blessings of a long life and vibrant, good health lasting right to the end of it. My research declares that this is fully achievable; I know that we can live every one of our days so blessed. I am committed to manifesting that future for myself and for each of my patients.

Through my practice, my fellow doctors in various fields of medicine, and from more alternative sources, I have steadily gathered data about the most effective anti-aging treatments, strategies, and methodologies available today. This book is the result. *By reading this book, you are embarking on a guided tour on the principles and practice on how to maintain and keep your health so you can age to perfection.*

My goal in writing Aged to Perfection is to clear the confusion about what will protect and enhance your maturing health. Our degrading ecosystem and the implications of greater longevity offer more complex challenges than previous generations have faced. So it is not surprising that, no matter how educated and motivated my patients are, the wealth of conflicting information is proved overwhelming.

In addition, recent breakthroughs in anti-aging medicine are helping to naturally, gently restore the energy and vigor of your youth without harmful side effects. You need to know about, for example, the bioidentical hormone therapy that can restore stability and balance throughout your body including your mind and emotions. This safe alternative is so much better than the cancer-causing synthetic hormones of bygone days. It is equally effective for male and female aging symptoms.

Through my patients, I know first-hand the satisfying results when this fully natural treatment is paired with a health-enhancing lifestyle. From impotence to premenstrual syndrome, to weight gain and sleeplessness, to the myriad symptoms of meno- and andropause, I have seen it all, and none of it must now be endured.

This is excellent news! It means that you can enjoy the wisdom and serenity that comes from maturity and the invigorating well being of bygone years. As a doctor, restoring health and preventing disease in such satisfying, natural ways drive my passion for preventive medicine.

It led to my medical degree, in 1983, from the Ohio University College of Osteopathic Medicine (Athens, Ohio). From its roots as a breakaway medical profession, it has experienced explosive growth throughout all fifty states. Founded in the early twentieth century, seeking healing modalities not found in traditional allopathic medicine of the day, osteopathic medicine combines the best of both worlds. It takes a whole-body (holistic), alternative approach to health, emphasizing the connection between the musculoskeletal system and disease, while utilizing all the diagnostic modalities, medications, and treatments that modern medicine has to offer.

This type of training naturally opened my mind to many types of healing. It also led to my keen interest in age-related disorders and becoming certified in Anti-Aging Medicine from the American Academy of Anti-Aging Medicine. I have utilized this, along with my companion certifications in Family Medicine and Emergency Medicine, and as an Independent Medical Examiner, to develop a holistic approach in my medical practice.

I am convinced that a person's entire body, mind, and spirit are intricately entwined in both the development of disease and the restoration of health. Through treating the whole person, a patient's biological clock can be reset to a time of greater vitality and youthfulness. This is truly inspiring because I have seen the heartbreaking consequences of an unhealthy lifestyle.

As director of Bellevue Hospital's emergency department (Ohio), where I also serve as assistant professor of emergency medicine for my alma mater, I constantly witness the anguish of loved ones as they struggle to deal with a life cut short because it was not lived in good health. I have pronounced the death of relatively young patients while my mind shouted that it was so needless. A commitment to small diet and lifestyle changes, supported by health-enhancing bioidentical hormones, could have extended that life by years or decades.

I think it is an utter tragedy that many people will live their last years, not in vibrant health but in misery, hindered by a poorly functioning body, drowning in despair, with skin prematurely aged, and life an endless round of medical appointments to treat completely preventable disorders. There is an alternative to this dreary picture.

No matter what your age, an optimal state of health and wellness can be reached with a health-enhancing lifestyle. The effects of aging are no longer to be tolerated, they are reversible. My holistic approach to anti-aging involves every facet of your life. You can expect to enjoy a rebalancing of your life so that it brings a deep, inner peace, a renewed enthusiasm for the adventure of living, and golden years of infinite goodness.

Running with the Bulls

Life is about enjoying each of its stages, embracing the lessons and enjoying the ride. I try to practice what I preach and ensure that I age gracefully, energetically, and realistically and enliven my life with positive experiences along the way.

As a young and, I must admit, less wise man, I flew to Pamplona, Spain with my brother for the sole purpose of running with the bulls in that city's annual event. It wasn't a sensible thing to do but I wanted to tap into my adventurous side; I wanted to do something I'd never done and to say I could do it.

Three shots were fired during the event; the third signals release of the bulls into the narrow, crowded streets. When I heard the third shot, I thought, "What on earth are we doing here?" Fear triggered an adrenal rush—not so much the fear of raging bulls but of getting trampled by all the drunkards staggering around me. It was tremendously exciting and unbelievably foolhardy.

Although with the wisdom of maturity I recognize the youthful recklessness behind that adventure, I also know that I could physically do the same again today because I have protected my health. I have plenty of adventures awaiting me as I look forward to my sixth decade on earth, and that is what makes my life truly worth living.

When you picture the later decades of your life, do you see yourself enjoying full, energetic days of marvelous exploration? Or do you choose as your birthright the sum total of an unhealthy way of living? In the latter case, you can expect pain, disease, and wearying days of immobility to be your dreary destiny. I don't accept that choice for myself. I hope you won't either. Together we will find a different way.

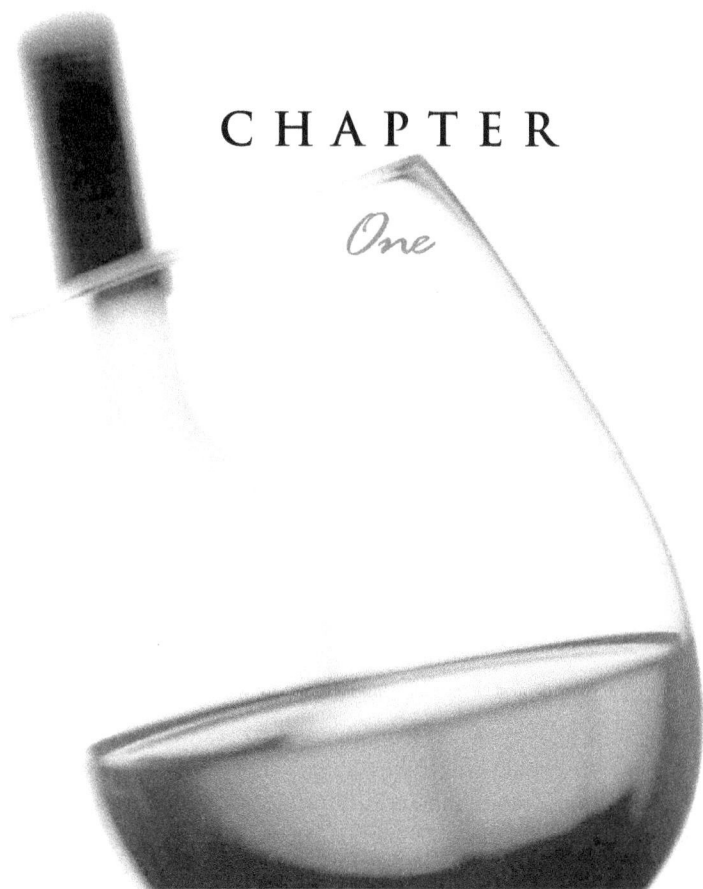

CHAPTER
One

CHAPTER ONE

Perfection in Your Prime

"It takes a long time to become young."

Pablo Picasso

My passion for aging with strength and vitality through the powers of the body, mind, and spirit is the driving force behind my writing. This combination of Western medicine and the time-tested wisdom of Eastern practices forms the philosophy that I have followed for years. However, it took a friend to say, "Roger, you have a book in you," to prompt me to put my thoughts into words.

I do not advocate seeking the Fountain of Youth because the bigger theme for this book, the great debate, so to speak, is that society may be obsessed with youth but it's quite okay not to be young. You've been through the wars of adolescence, raising a family, and contributing to society, so you've earned the wisdom that is reflected in your eyes and face. If you have sagging skin and wrinkles, these are your battle scars and you should wear them with pride.

There are advantages to every stage of life. Where you are now is the result of countless invaluable lessons learned from decades of dealing with this planet and its inhabitants, creating a foundation for the outlook you have today. If regrets or dissatisfying relationships are currently marring your point of view, read on: this book is not just about physical health but holistic wellness throughout your body, mind, and spirit.

Just as a flawless diamond is forged through incredible heat and pressure, the confidence and competence of your later years are the products of being tested and honed by the challenges experienced in your youth. Life lessons, well learned, serve to transform the brash arrogance of the immature into the confidence and poise that is so often the greatest beauty in a face no longer young.

In fact, most people would not want to go back to their youth, despite what the media says and its alluring depictions of youth. It is such a fleeting stage in life! When it leaves, although the freshness of youth may go, gone too are the juvenile insecurities that stem from a lack of experience and shallow self-understanding.

Be comfortable with your age. This doesn't mean you can't feel great, especially if you are struggling with age-related issues such as fatigue, weight gain, mental confusion, mood swings, or sexual problems. This book is about resolving these issues so that you can enjoy the rewards of maturity without the ill health that may often accompany it.

Aging gracefully, actively, and vibrantly means that you can continue to move easily, think with clarity, be sexually and socially active, maintain the optimism and zest of youth, and feel comfortable dealing with your life and relationships. By following the proven wisdom and innovative therapies in this book, you can ensure that this will be your future. Don't let it be the prospect of painful arthritis and debilitating diseases, mental confusion or dementia, and other life-sapping conditions such that you can't enjoy yourself and spend the last 20 years of your life immobilized in a dreary nursing home.

My own mid-life revelation, which occurred at a convention of the American Academy of Anti-Aging Medicine, helped me to understand how a natural, holistic approach to medicine would click with my philosophy of wellness. It set me on a new career path.

I had the opportunity to train with Dr. Paul Savage, founder of BodyLogicMD, who was featured in Suzanne Somers' 2006 book, *Ageless,* and is one of the great minds in anti-aging medicine. I learned a tremendous amount about using diet, natural supplements, bioidentical hormones, and healthy living habits to rejuvenate a mature person's life and resolve chronic ailments that have been sapping his or her vitality and youthful outlook. Now my life purpose is to help my patients, know how to age wholly, naturally, and gracefully.

My desire is that you choose to come with me on a journey of discovery. It is a choice because it involves a willingness to do what it takes to improve your life. What I have learned about preserving youthful vitality and wellness throughout the aging process will, I hope, educate and inspire you to nurture your life on every level.

You can protect and enhance the quality of life you enjoy with preventive, holistic medicine. Read this book at leisure; highlight what pops out at you, flip to a topic that grabs you, and read on. I guarantee that nourishing your powerful body-mind-soul connection will help you to age with optimal vitality and wellness.

The Rock Doc

You can reap huge benefits in wellness by making simple but powerful changes to your lifestyle. The goal is to achieve balance on all levels. If you aren't convinced this is necessary, just think of yourself as a rock star.

Based on positive results with my patients and some magical, word-of-mouth recommendations, I was given the opportunity to work with several traveling celebrities, eventually earning the moniker "The Rock Doc." The experience was a real eye-opener on the rigors of an unhealthy lifestyle: relentless stress, social isolation, indulgence in addictive activities, and an on-the-go, sub-optimal diet.

These artists were dealing with problems related to low stamina, chronic pain, high blood pressure, and sleep deprivation, among other ailments. Does this sound familiar? There are worrisome parallels between this lifestyle and that of a typical stressed-out Baby Boomer whose schedule leaves no time for healthy eating, sleeping, and playing.

Many people revere the rock star life but the harsh reality is far from glamorous. Star-struck fans may think a celebrity's life is charmed, pampered, and problem free, but their lives are far worse than average. These artists, who are on the road all the time, are cut off from everything that constitutes a holistic and healthy lifestyle. They are surrounded by multiple temptations, such as plentiful drugs and alcohol, and loveless, empty sexual encounters. The latter, which offer little emotional support, compound the problem by causing isolation from their friends and loved ones.

In most cases, they needed to boost their immune systems, so I used supplements and, in some cases, Vitamin B12 injections to help them feel better and have more energy. Not surprisingly, some entertainers have the worst diets on the planet, so nutritional advice was a significant component of their treatment. I have no celebrity lust because they are talented but imperfect human beings who need help just like the rest of us. Their health equally benefits from guidance on the factors that go into a wellness lifestyle.

The Vitality Factors

The following vitality factors are essential for ensuring a robustly healthy, strong, and vigorous future. My research identifies these factors as powerful components that interconnect to activate all levels of your body-mind-spirit connection. How this happens will be discussed in detail in later chapters.

Bioidentical hormones. Through Dr. Savage, and the American Academy of Anti-Aging Medicine, I have documented how the steady decline of critical hormones leads to a complex array of debilitating ailments. It is important to realize that this situation must be reversed if you want to remain vigorously healthy with a sharp intellect and youthful appearance. Bioidentical hormones are the solution; they act holistically throughout the body without causing harmful side effects.

Available since the 1930s, these natural, plant-sourced supplements are compounded from plant extracts and exactly replicate human hormones. They protect a person's health in innumerable ways by restoring hormone levels and helping to prevent disease. Bioidentical hormones are effective without the risks, such as cancer, that are associated with synthetic hormones made from potentially harmful ingredients like pregnant mares' urine.

In addition, recent innovations in application techniques have maximized the delivery of these hormones to the body. They include subcutaneous pellets, topical patches, and creams. See chapter 3 for an in-depth discussion of hormone health and the powerfully rejuvenating effects of bioidentical hormones.

Although the research and use of natural, bioidentical hormones have been well documented for years, only in the last decade has this knowledge spread to the general public. If you are old enough to remember the fears and controversy related to using acupuncture in North America 30 years ago, it will give you an idea of how long it takes to educate and inform both consumers and Western doctors about the safety of an alternative treatment.

We can thank advocates like Suzanne Somers for getting the word out to everyday people on their benefits. Somers devotes much of her book, *Ageless*, to bioidentical hormones. As a further boost in public education, in 2009, the Oprah Winfrey show included three separate segments on bioidentical hormones.

Choosing to change. Your attitude is important; wanting to change is an important factor in opening yourself up to the possibilities. If you want to feel robustly healthy from now on, you must be willing to do what it takes to realize this goal.

Visualize the kind of life you want to lead and commit to doing what it takes to achieve this vision on every level. Choose to begin creating a wellness lifestyle that will keep you constantly feeling absolutely marvelous.

Small, steady advances. If you're not happy with being you, it's never too late to change and live the life you've always wanted. It takes some effort, but it won't take a marathon, a nutritionist, or an expensive program to maximize your age and wellness. Simply by steadily making small changes, you can improve how you feel and how your body functions, and you can even extend your life.

Small things will add up to make a tremendous difference in your overall health. You don't need to spend a lot of money, but you must commit to a steady, step-by-step progression in your transformation to absolute wellness.

For example, physical exercise is a key factor in wellness but you don't have to join an expensive gym or begin marathon training. You can start by walking around the block during your lunch hour and get a dose of Vitamin D at the same time. This simple exercise will affect your body-mind-spirit connection. Experienced psychologists will often kick-start therapy with their patients by recommending daily exercise to boost their natural feel-good hormones and reduce depression.

This simple step can literally change your life. Making small changes is also less stressful because it is a gradual process. As we will discuss, stress is another major factor in how you grow older. You don't need to add more stress by placing huge expectations on yourself as you seek to improve your health.

Physical health and hormones. The foundation of body-mind-spirit wholeness is physical balance because it profoundly impacts your moods, emotions, and overall outlook. Physical well-being includes the body boosts of nutrition, nutraceutical supplementation, bioidentical hormones, and consistent exercise. Strategies to minimize the effects of our toxic environment are also important.

When it comes to nutrition, you can learn to make simpler choices and strive for a whole-food, plant-based diet more frequently. We are all busy and we all like to eat out for convenience, but stop doing it so often. This simple change will offer dividends in reducing weight and eliminating hidden toxins.

As you will see in upcoming chapters, the use of nutraceutical supplements can quickly change how you feel for an encouraging jump-start to your wellness. The recommended daily allowance of many vitamins is not enough to prevent degenerative changes and the foods we eat are often suboptimal in nutrients. Certain supplements also offer other health benefits. What to take, and how much to take, will be covered in chapter 4.

Positive living. To enjoy each stage of your life, your attitude is critical. If you wallow in past regrets or endure ongoing unpleasantness in your relationships, your zest for life will be affected. In our time-stressed culture, you can overlook the requirement to feed your spirit; developing a positive attitude makes a tremendous difference. It will determine, for example, if you believe that the changes we're discussing in this book are even possible for you.

Living with an unhealthy relationship is a huge factor that affects wellness at any age. Yet old, emotional wounds are often shoved into a dark corner of the mind in the hope they will fade like a lost memory. Unfortunately, avoiding the issue will often create the opposite effect: uncontrollable bursts of anger, impatience, fatigue, or depression.

Positive changes leapfrog into other areas of life and can be unexpected. I get calls from patients at odd hours, who often say things like, "Dr. Garcia, I've patched my relationship with my daughter. It's wonderful!" After receiving that impromptu call from a patient, I knew the healing with her daughter had changed both of them so radically that the next step is wellness.

Small changes include healing the relationships with your closest loved ones. If you didn't have the perfect relationship with your mother or father, for example, perhaps it's time to make a small step to mend it. It will probably reap dividends for the rest of your life.

Get support. When making permanent lifestyle changes, many people benefit from having someone supportive provide encouragement and motivation. Often I function as a physical exercise coach as well as an anti-aging coach. Others use the buddy system to help each other in their quest to change.

If this applies to you, then get support from a friend or professional as you develop your anti-aging lifestyle. Isolation does not suit you: we are inherently social creatures, needing meaningful interactions with others for happiness. Studies indicate that older adults who live lonely, disconnected lives are more vulnerable to cognitive impairment conditions such as Alzheimer's disease, dementia, and depression, in addition to many chronic diseases.

Active stress reduction. Stress is a killer. It literally eats your physical brain. In our time-stressed, overworked, fast-changing world, stress is unavoidable, and how you manage stress is an increasingly important factor as you age.

You need an ongoing stress-busting component to your life, such as breathing techniques, massage, yoga, meditation, or exercise, because it affects the body-mind-spirit connection in multiple ways. For example, reducing stress improves your energy and hormone levels. It enhances feelings of peace in your life, which improves your mood. It reduces feelings of distractedness and increases awareness of what's going on in your world.

How do you deal with stress? The simplest stress-buster is achieved through deep breathing techniques. Slow, steady breathing is a huge de-stressor. The relaxing technique of deep breathing can be done in your car during rush hour, on the subway, in a line-up, and virtually anywhere. It's a great help for managing stressful situations.

Keeping the World Young

My passions include encouraging people to embrace the power of the body, mind, and spirit and promoting a world standard of wellness. I have now found my calling in life. I wanted to become a doctor to help people heal in every way, not just physically. With a holistic approach to anti-aging medicine, I can finally say that I am accomplishing this for my patients.

It excites me every day. An unexpected result of following my passion is the doors that are opening for me to educate people about preventing disease and remaining youthful. I closely identify with people who have been ostracized by the traditional medical community and I try even harder to reassure them that there is help. The rewards have been countless.

The advice in the following chapters is based on trusted research and evidence-based studies; it embraces the use of all modalities to slow down age-related decline. It also examines the root cause of age-related illness and the treatments necessary to alleviate them.

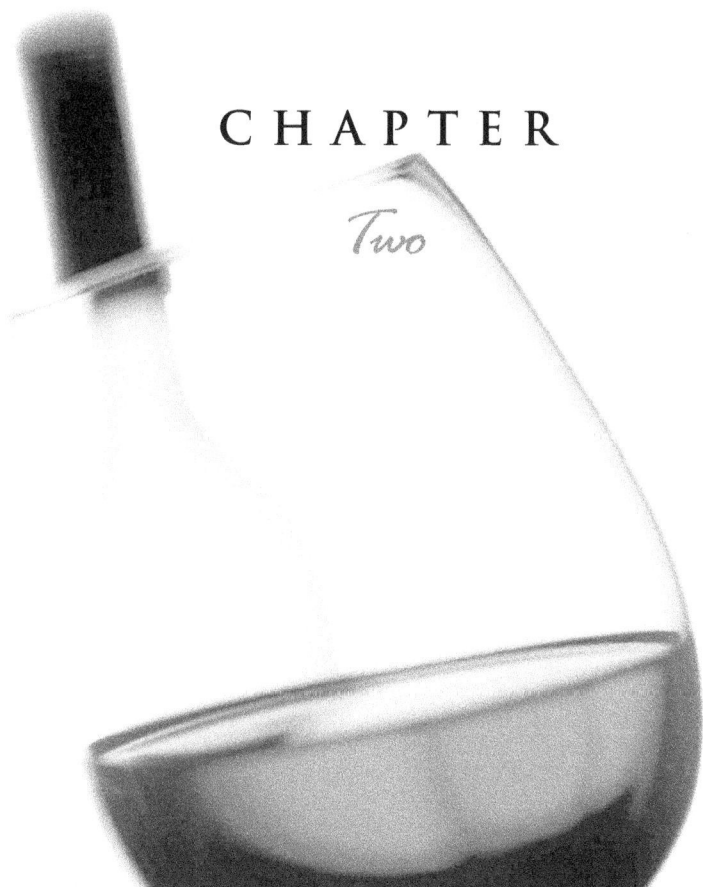

CHAPTER

Two

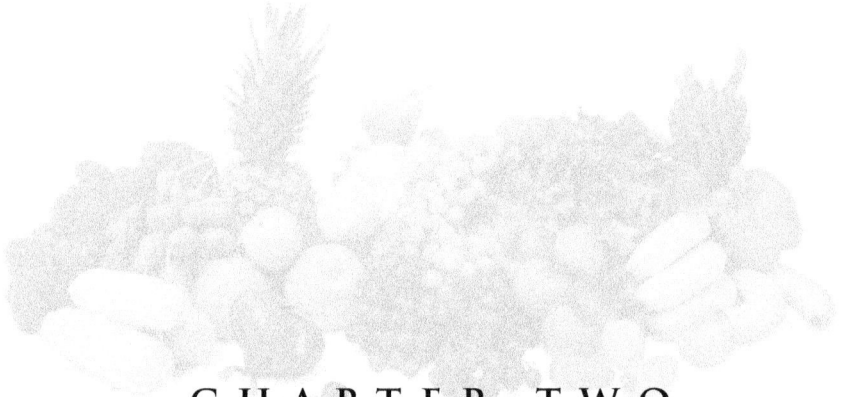

CHAPTER TWO

A New Beginning

"Age is opportunity no less
Than youth itself, though in another dress,
And as the evening twilight fades away
The sky is filled with stars, invisible by day."

Henry Wordsworth Longfellow,
Morituri Salutamus

D o you feel the way you used to? Or has your life changed because a series of ailments is leaving you feeling "off" and older that you want to feel? However healthy you are, and regardless of your physical condition, you can begin your return to a youthful state of glowing vitality right now: it's never too late!

The symptoms of aging vary from one person to the next, covering a wide spectrum, but the following will give you a good, general idea. Physically, you might have low energy or sexual drive, headaches or migraines, unexplained aches and pains, weight gain (especially around the middle) that you have unsuccessfully tried to control, muscle weakness, insomnia, hot flashes or night sweats, and bone loss, among other symptoms. Men may also experience impotence, while women may experience vaginal dryness and pain during intercourse. Mentally, there may be fuzzy thinking, confusion, or an inability to remember anything from a word in mid-sentence to why you were going upstairs. Emotionally, you may have wild mood swings or you may experience depression, anger, or anxiety.

Your zest for life will probably be lacking, which is not surprising considering all the issues you're dealing with. *Aged to Perfection* is about creating a vigorous routine of health that will reverse the types of symptoms mentioned above. Your body is amazingly resilient! It will respond to every change you make, the sum of which will lead to a dramatic improvement in your health and enthusiasm for life.

But first, you have to get the ball rolling. Recovering what you once had will take some concentrated effort and a conscious decision to act. The old cliché that we get set in our ways carries more than a grain of truth. Most people resist change, and as we mature we become very comfortable with our own pace, diet, lifestyle, and bad habits. But change is the only thing that will get back your life.

Small, steady improvements can turn your body clock back many decades. A positive change in one area of life acts like a magnet to attract more improvements. I've seen it work for so many people that I'm convinced this is the route back to improved health.

Sometimes, kick-starting change requires a nudge from a doctor like me. I'm just a glorified life coach; my patients do the work, but I help them to get started. Then something magical happens, deep inside them. After that, my role is to encourage them to keep going. If you feel that you'd benefit from ongoing encouragement, then by all means get it; invest in your vibrantly healthy future. Using a coach, or a good buddy system, will help anyone to excel at reaching his or her goals. That's the foundation of all coaching, even the peer coaching that we call the buddy system.

Getting back into balance by activating the body-mind-spirit connection is your key to achieving powerful vitality and robust enthusiasm for life. In this chapter, you will read about people who have struggled with health challenges that may sound painfully familiar. But they each triumphed and so can you, if you want it bad enough.

Managing the Unmanageable

Rhonda Andretti, age 56, began experiencing the symptoms of menopause shortly after her 50th birthday. They included hot flashes, mood swings, anxiety, night sweats, sleeplessness, fatigue, fuzzy thinking, itching, vaginal dryness and pain during intercourse, and complete loss of libido.

As she says, "I had them all! Every symptom of menopause known to man. I tried all the over-the-counter remedies but none of them worked for me. I didn't want to take synthetic hormone replacement therapy due to the fear of cancer, but my life had become so unmanageable that I felt like I had no choice." Her gynecologist prescribed synthetic estrogen. The hot flashes, night sweats, and sleeplessness began to subside in a few weeks, but she still experienced severe anxiety, irritability, and poor libido.

Her life had become a living hell at a time when she needed to feel good about her increasing maturity. "I had lost my zest for life. I had also lost my daughter in a tragic car accident and was raising her young children. The death of a child is devastating, but added to this was the full responsibility for two beautiful little girls who had just lost their mother, and a demanding career, all topped off with these menopause symptoms. There were times when I thought I was losing my mind."

So her doctor prescribed an antidepressant. "Talk about losing your love of life: it made me lethargic and miserable. I didn't want to go anywhere or do anything. I would lose my temper with the children and then cry because I knew they didn't deserve my impatience and irritability. My husband tried to be supportive and help but just couldn't understand what I was going through."

Two hours from her home, she found me in Columbus, Ohio. As she describes it, "That day, I started on the journey to get my life back. I am now on bioidentical hormones that address all of my symptoms, as well as some nutritional supplements. I am now sleeping and the hot flashes and night sweats have disappeared. My libido is better. But most importantly, I am no longer so quick to anger or constantly irritable. I have patience with my two girls and life is more harmonious. The joy has returned to my life."

This kind of return to wholeness and optimism is very gratifying. The nutritional supplements, or nutraceuticals, helped to speed her return to excellent health. Her treatment with natural, bioidentical hormones, which are free of side effects, relieved all her menopausal symptoms and restored a balanced feeling of vitality on many levels.

Hormonal imbalances are a common hallmark of aging. Unaddressed, they sap your physical health and steal your enthusiasm for living. They can also cause major illnesses such as cancer. Bioidentical hormones have the same molecular structure as the hormones produced naturally within your body. This enables them to be properly utilized and naturally metabolized to restore the body's balance. They can actually protect you from harmful diseases while acting holistically to repair the strength and verve that often goes missing as we mature.

Bioidentical hormones helped to restore Rhonda's quality of life on every level: physically, emotionally, and mentally. That's the whole-body effect of these plant-based supplements. The results can be nothing short of incredible, especially when combined with other wellness practices such as regular exercise and improved nutrition. For more information on how they work and the benefits you can expect, read chapter 3.

The Right Kind of Change

The following story is another example of the desperation and hopelessness that many people face. It will inspire you with the all-encompassing, potent return to health that is very possible. My proven approach helped Robert Herald to recapture the vital energy and glowing constitution eroded by time.

How he regained his vitality and youthful enthusiasm will encourage you to accomplish the same in your life.

At age 46, Robert had high blood pressure and needed to lose more than 50 pounds. His blood tests indicated too little good cholesterol and too much of the bad kind. He said that he was constantly tired, was nearly impotent, had very little sex drive, and could barely concentrate at work, which was beginning to affect his job. His efforts to counteract the effects of aging were unproductive. He had tried to lose weight with a drastic, reduced-calorie diet but it only aggravated his symptoms and left him constantly hungry.

Repeated attempts to get help from doctors had been unsuccessful. As he describes it, "I would end up with another new prescription for some type of drug with all kinds of possible scary side effects and the necessity to take regular blood tests to make sure they weren't causing liver damage. I was on two cholesterol meds, two blood pressure meds, two meds for gout for which I had frequent attacks, a synthetic for my thyroid, and a prescription for Viagra that I rarely had to refill because I really didn't have much interest anyway."

He came to me to discuss what he called andropause-related hormone deficiencies, and was pleased with the treatment protocol. "I was very surprised to spend so much time talking to Dr. Garcia and not have him speeding out the door while handing me another prescription for some chemical. We went over the blood test, line by line, and he made recommendations to improve those not-so-good areas."

We discussed some dietary supplements to improve his cholesterol problem. I prescribed bioidenticals, including testosterone, progesterone, and Armour Thyroid, which is more natural than the drug Robert was taking. The effects of this treatment, in combination with his determination to get strong and healthy, satisfied both of us.

One year later, he reported many improvements. He had more muscle and less body fat. A diet based on six small, daily meals of fresh, organic foods instead of processed, fast foods led to a weight loss of 52 pounds. He says that he is never hungry because "I basically eat all day: the good stuff." Before, any exercise was painful because it aggravated a back injury, but this quickly turned around. With the weight loss his pain disappeared; so did the aggravating gout. He took up running as well as riding his bike about 20 miles, twice a week. He is looking forward to starting weight training soon. "This would have been impossible for me a year ago," he says.

His overall vitality improved tremendously. "I have a sex life again with no need for Viagra. My blood pressure today is normal and I am completely off cholesterol meds." Robert says his concentration and general mood are both improved. "I'm not so grouchy all the time. I'm feeling more motivated than ever and have started enjoying hobbies like hiking, fishing, and treasure hunting, which I used to love but had lost energy for. People who haven't seen me in a while are amazed. They ask me if I went on a diet and I tell them no, it's a life-extension program."

A recent stress test and heart echo indicated he now has less than a one percent chance of having a heart attack. "This is great news since both my parents have had heart bypasses and several angioplasties." His example proves that our genetic "risk factors," as doctors call them, comprise only 25 percent of our destiny. The rest is wholly under our control.

A Desperate Life

I recently visited the fascinating, traveling display Bodies...The Exhibition, which features actual human specimens and graphically depicts all that goes on underneath our skin. The philosophy behind this exhibit was scrolled in large letters across the wall beside the exit. In essence, it said that it often takes a life-threatening event, when we're flat on our backs and forced to reflect, to fully appreciate the healthy body and mind that we often take for granted.

Desperation or illness is often the catalyst for change in our lives. A dramatic downturn in health can be the only thing that drives us to seek answers. In our fast-food, quick-fix society, the concerted effort required for a long-term solution may seem very unappealing. Sadly, once a person recovers from an illness or surgery, that short-lived memory often fades and he or she reverts to old, unhealthy habits.

In a small percentage of people, fear is successful at engendering long-term changes, but the majority don't react this way. Dr. Edward Miller, dean of the medical school at Johns Hopkins University, reported a study in which, two years after having major heart surgery, 90 percent of people had not changed their lifestyle.

On the other hand, the Preventative Medicine Research Institute in Sausalito, California, reported a 77 percent success rate in heart patients' ability to maintain lifestyle changes over three years. The difference was a year of twice-weekly, group-support sessions and instruction in meditation, relaxation, yoga, and aerobic exercise. This steady, long-term support brought about a lasting life transformation.

Regarding his study, Dr. Dean Ornish, professor of medicine at University of California (San Francisco), said that motivating people through fear of dying was much less effective than helping them to find the joy of living by convincing them that they can feel better, and not just live longer. He recommended treatment that would "bring in the psychological, emotional, and spiritual dimensions that are so often ignored." This body-mind-spirit connection is your most powerful tool for reviving youthful vigor.

You must make a commitment to changing how you live; if you need ongoing support to do this, then by all means, get it. I emphasize baby steps to aging optimally because this results in permanent, lasting change. If you fall off the wagon, just hop on board again the next day. Don't beat yourself up. It's never too late!

You are not alone in dealing with the effects of an aging body. We are in the midst of an exploding "epidemic" of aging because of the Baby Boomer effect. This group of people, roughly 50 to 65 years of age, is a post-war, demographic bulge and most of them are now bulging physically. Americans in their sixties include two recent presidents, George W. Bush and Bill Clinton, and well-known celebrities Cher, Donald Trump, Sylvester Stallone, and Dolly Parton.

Born into an era of tremendous prosperity, conveniences poured off manufacturers' production lines at unprecedented rates. From fast foods to technology, most of these comforts had unhealthy side effects. The quality of their life began to suffer as a result and nothing short of a complete lifestyle change can reverse the damage.

Time Out

Stress and overwork are killers. I know that workaholics don't want to hear this, but believe me, they are deadly. Stress is responsible for the rapid acceleration of aging; I will detail its life-damaging effects in chapter 5. If you deal with unremitting pressure and demands, your return to health could start with carving out some "you" time every day. It could literally save your life.

Robin McGraw, Dr. Phil's wife, is a wonderful advocate for taking care of oneself. She walks the talk. Every day, Robin blocks off an hour in her schedule for her time. Her family knows that she is not to be disturbed unless it's an emergency. She has a number of wellness techniques that nourish her body, mind, and soul and relishes the time to turn off the busy demands in her life. This daily habit is now so engrained in Robin's schedule that it's as automatic and beneficial as brushing her teeth every day.

Retreating from all the pressure into smart, life-protecting strategies is proven to yield significant dividends. When it comes to dramatic change from taking time out, I can't think of a better example than Joe Stanton, a rural pastor in Ohio who was withdrawn and suicidal at our first meeting. His wife accompanied him, and she told me in confidence that I was her last chance before she would have to take him to a psychiatric institution because he was so dangerously depressed.

Over a period of several months, he had changed from a lively, active, engaging gentleman into someone who was withdrawn and suicidal. His story reflects the constant strain that so many of us endure daily. Unremitting demands from tending the needs of his flock included two to three religious services per week and countless hospital visits, personal counseling, and funerals.

As a doctor, I find that many stressed patients are so focused on keeping going that sometimes you have to give them permission to stop. What they need to hear from someone with authority (such as a doctor) is that it's okay to take time off. They can be their own worst enemy; they beat themselves up for feeling how they do but we all need time off from the pressures of our increasingly hectic world. We need it for the good of our health.

Joe had neglected himself until he was completely debilitated and forced to take a six-month leave from his vocation. Friends, alarmed when they saw him, recommended me and he began a "miraculous recovery to life," as he calls it. Within four to five months, he came around very quickly and his family and friends could not believe the dramatic change.

Joe describes the incredibly damaged man I first saw. "Stress, fatigue, and over-commitment, combined with age, were taking a toll on my body, soul, and mind, not to mention my wife and family. Chronic fatigue, depression, sleeplessness, and the inability to think clearly made it necessary for me to take some time off." His symptoms also included heart rhythm irregularities, insomnia, weight gain despite a loss of appetite, and no libido.

Forced to retreat into self-care his life depended on, we discussed the effects of unrelenting stress. "I had no idea that very high cortisol levels and extremely low progesterone and testosterone were the primary culprits in my rapid regression from life," he says. I treated him with bioidentical hormones and nutritional supplements, and helped him to understand the damaging effects of unhealthy eating.

"I began to come back to life again. My mind began to clear, the depression lifted, chronic fatigue was replaced by energy and a renewed zest for life, and the sleeplessness was gone," he says. "With the increased energy levels I could begin a regular exercise routine again, and actually began building lean muscle mass and losing a very stubborn layer of abdominal fat that had been building for a number of years." During the next two years, his weight dropped by 30 pounds.

Bioidentical testosterone helped; it was a major component in his recovery. It has a holistic effect on many of the body's functions and also lifts depression. But for Joe, talking to him helped a lot. It gave him permission to begin paying a bit more attention to himself. For over-dedicated people like Joe, it's the difference between life and death

Two months later, he returned to his life's calling and a newly active lifestyle. "My wife, my children, and my grandchildren were thrilled to see me emerge from my 'dark night of the soul.' I was alive again." His renewed drive to exercise, and engage life head on, meant that "daily life and a busy, demanding schedule are no longer draining the life from me. The stress levels of my vocation have not diminished, but my capacity to deal with all the demands greatly increased." His stress strategy includes "morning prayer and meditation, a regular stretching routine, and a good combination of aerobic and weight-bearing exercises."

Joe also follows a program of healthy, nutritious eating. "Along with my supplements, my bioidentical hormone replacement therapy will be a part of my daily routine and life from now on. It all adds up to a brand new me!"

Healing Touches

In each of these stories, my most important role as a doctor has been encouraging my patients to thrive. Treating someone like Rhonda with a prescription antidepressant, or loading patients with "chemicals" as Robert described, will not produce a return to health. As a doctor, it is my responsibility to not only act as a guide on what can return my patient to good health but also encourage him or her along the way.

Small gestures such as a kind word or gentle touch will make a tremendous difference in people's lives and moods. It's hard to teach empathy and compassion, and most doctors have had this beaten out of them after years of training and being in the trenches. They've lost it. Part of my work as director of the emergency department at Bellevue Hospital is hiring doctors. I will pass on hiring some of the best-trained doctors because they don't have the compassion to make things work in our emergency room.

In my family, we never shied away from saying we loved each other. It taught me that kind, empathetic words heal and uplift our spirits and sometimes produce magical results. I vividly remember a patient who was being flown out for emergency surgery after suffering a severe heart attack. He was in critical condition and I didn't know if he was going to make it. While he was lying on the stretcher, I leaned down to the man and whispered, "I will think of you in my prayers tonight."

As soon as I said these words, something happened to him that I couldn't explain. There was a visible shift. What I can say for certain is the power of the mind-body-spirit connection was firing on all cylinders. The patient survived the flight and his open-heart surgery. The first words he uttered when he regained consciousness were what I had said to him.

As an emergency room doctor, I've seen a lot of death because I encounter so many people during their last moments. I've listened to the wailings of family members whose father has just had a massive heart attack, and I've had to tell parents that I cannot save the life of their 14-year-old son. If that doesn't affect you, then nothing will. This is my background and it has taught me the true power of kindness, compassion, and healing touches.

I'd rather have an average doctor with good interpersonal skills and empathy than a doctor who is superior but lacking in this area. That's how critically important I've found these qualities to be.

Most of us realize that our society does not have a very affectionate culture, and yet touch is vital for our well-being. Touching shows a little compassion for another person's situation, but most doctors won't touch a patient. As a doctor, touch is one of the most common things that helps people. When I have to give bad news, I'm usually touching a patient's forehead or shoulder. It's something so simple, yet it is such a tremendous healing technique. Touch is a means of communication so critical that its absence retards growth in infants. It is a long-noted syndrome that infants deprived of direct human contact grow slowly and even die.

In my practice, patients will often instinctively hug me before they leave my office. My secretary, who sees other doctors' patients leave the clinic, said to me one day, "I don't see other doctors at the clinic getting a hug from their patients." Sharing hugs is not something I set out to do, it just happens; it's innate and it's wonderful to see the way it reassures and inspires people.

I was nurtured by parents in a traditional, religious upbringing: a very close-knit, physically affectionate family. My father is 88 years old and I still hug him and kiss him every time I see him. It's natural for me to reach out in this way, and it has many health benefits. For both men and women, I highly recommend adopting a regular practice of hugging.

A good hug is a quick, anti-stress remedy, as spiritually healing as hours of meditation. Regular touch establishes a connection between your body, mind, and spirit and has been proven to decrease anxiety, elevate white blood cell counts, lower blood pressure, increase the level of feel-good endorphins, and help you sleep better.

A team from the University of North Carolina, studying the effects of hugging, determined that hugs increased the levels of oxytocin, a "bonding" hormone, and reduced blood pressure, which cuts the risk of heart disease. No wonder it's so good to get and receive hugs.

As a doctor, I need to listen carefully to my patients, discover their symptoms, and then develop a personalized therapy program. As a man, I need to encourage them along the journey back to health, with a kind word and sometimes with a nice, big hug.

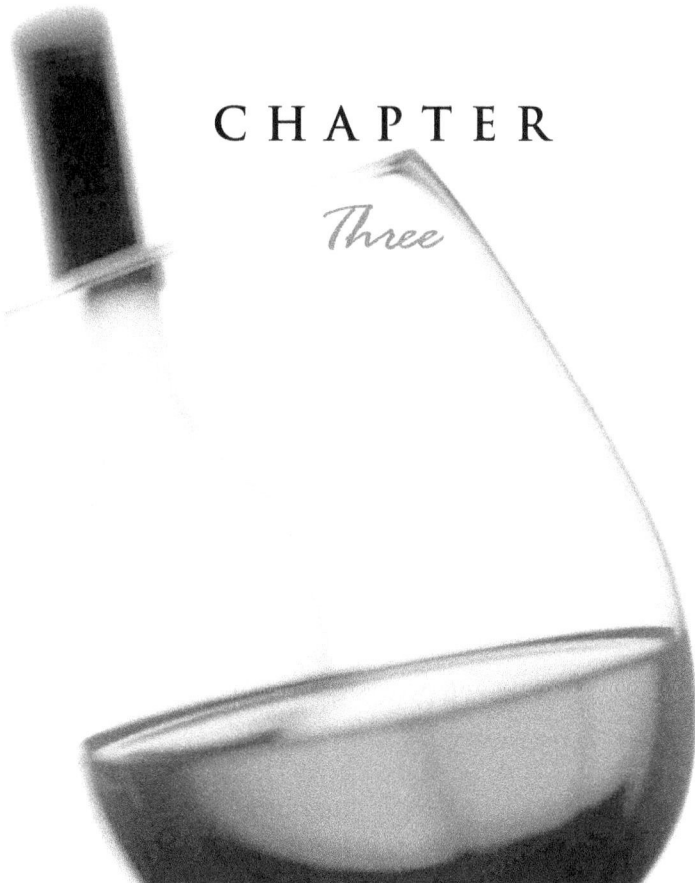

CHAPTER

Three

CHAPTER THREE

Your Body Renewed

"The Lord hath created medicines out of the earth;
and he that is wise will not abhor them."

E c c l e s i a s t i c u s   3 8 : 4

When it comes to the subject of synthetic and bioidentical hormones, I'm going to jump right in and dispel some of the myths surrounding this hot topic. There is no shortage of misinformation, confusion, and fear; synthetic hormones are the cause of all the distress. For more than 30 years, natural, bioidentical hormones have been used with minimal side effects; in fact, they even protect against diseases such as cancer. That's why I prescribe them, and I've seen exciting successes in my patients.

For decades, women were prescribed drugs such as Premarin, a synthetic estrogen produced from the urine of pregnant mares. Then, in 2002, to the disbelief and alarm of countless women and their doctors, the Women's Health Initiative (WHI) abruptly stopped its major study of synthetic estrogen three years early. Preliminary results indicated a disquieting increase in breast cancer, blood clots, and stroke from using these synthetic drugs. The shockwave among millions of women caused roughly 50 percent to discontinue, or reduce, their dosage of these virulent, artificial drugs, which I call "alien" drugs because they do not exist naturally in the human body nor on Earth (they are chemically altered hormones conceived in the laboratory by Big Pharma to secure a patent).

Many turned to herbal remedies with limited success. Others, deprived of this measly, partial solution to their symptoms, sighed and continued to suffer.

Some traditional doctors suggested that synthetic and bioidentical hormones have the same dire side effects, but that's not the case at all. The news reports made no distinction between synthetic drugs and natural, bioidentical estrogen, which was not studied at all. This is a huge point. Much of this book is aimed at clearing up misconceptions about synthetic and bioidentical hormones.

So here's the short answer: for more than 30 years, doctors like me have been prescribing bioidentical hormones with minimal observable side effects, In addition, they have been found to be very protective against cancer and other chronic diseases. That's how powerfully health-enhancing these natural, plant-based medicines are. Hormone imbalance is a devastatingly real part of growing older and bioidentical hormones provide a safe, whole-body solution that works.

I must add, though, that this book is not about bashing traditional doctors and medicine. Everyone's different, and in some cases pharmaceutical drugs are necessary to support a patient on the journey back to truly vibrant, youthful vitality. For example, I've used blood pressure medications to treat the celebrities I described in chapter 1, and Robert Herald (from chapter 2) had to remain on this medication until his weight dropped and his health improved enough for him to be rid of them.

In a perfect world, traditional and alternative practitioners would support and complement each other to their patients' benefit. It could provide more choices in health care. Nonetheless, more men and women are seeking natural solutions to restoring hormonal balance, and that's where doctors of holistic, preventive medicine come in. Today's consumers are discovering the benefits of bioidentical hormones, so the word is getting out.

Time-Tested and Safe

Bioidentical hormones have the same molecular structure as the hormones produced naturally in our bodies. Because of their identical chemical structure, they are effectively processed, utilized, and excreted. All bioidentical hormones originate from Mexican wild yam, plant sterols, or soybeans. The technique that turns these plants into a compound, with the identical structure to our body's hormones, was discovered in the 1930s.

Pennsylvania State University professor Russell Marker extracted the steroid precursor chemical diosgenin from the Mexican yam *(Dioscorea composita)*, which grew wild around my birthplace in the state of Veracruz, Mexico. He was able to transform this wild yam into natural bioidentical progesterone. The development of this innovative treatment, has revolutionized the experience of aging for millions of people. One of most effective forms of natural, bioidentical progesterone is called micronized progesterone USP. It is produced under rigorous quality standards, it allows for steady and even absorption by the body, and it is only available through a doctor's prescription.

Natural progesterone creams are also available over the counter. Both prescription and commercial types of cream contain varying amounts of bioidentical progesterone. However, when using any medication it is important to obtain the advice of a trusted medical practitioner. Everyone is different, and what is appropriate for one person may not work for another.

When your hormones get back into balance, the effect is a whole-body harmony and a recapturing of the energy and glowing constitution of your youth. Getting there isn't a hit-and-miss progression but an individualized process. It starts with lab tests to measure the level of several hormones such as estrogen, testosterone, progesterone, and cortisol. Thyroid studies measure the two thyroid hormones, T3 and T4 (for an overview of these two hormones, read "Thyroid Traumas" in this chapter). Other tests profile your current health, which include measuring blood-sugar metabolism, cholesterol levels, and other biomarkers of aging.

At the same time, I also listen carefully to my patient, noting symptoms and evaluating the state of his or her health, diet, and fitness regime. When I finally prescribe bioidentical hormones, it is within an overall treatment protocol that includes nutraceutical supplements and guidance on critical diet and lifestyle changes.

People might think that bioidentical hormones are part of the trend toward natural, alternative medicine. But they have been produced commercially on a large scale for more than 30 years, as they include Estrace tablets and certain vaginal creams, estrogen skin patches, topical gels, and pellets. They are not new to the marketplace, and studies on bioidentical hormones have been around for many years.

However, there has been increased interest in hormones because of the health threats now associated with synthetic hormone drugs. Typically, it takes an average of 25 years for new ideas to be included as state-of-the art medicine. So, when it comes to research and hands-on results, this time-lag effect has brought bioidentical hormones into perfect alignment with modern preferences.

This type of time lag has occurred with other treatments. For example, in 1982, the discovery that stomach and duodenal ulcers were caused by the bacterium *Helicobacter pylori* was considered absolute heresy at the time. Stress and lifestyle were considered the key causes of ulcers. Two Australian scientists, Barry J. Marshall and J. Robin Warren, discovered this link but were ridiculed by their medical colleagues. Years later, in 2005, these innovative scientists received the Nobel Prize in Physiology or Medicine for their groundbreaking discovery that peptic ulcers were an infectious disease! Before this research was accepted, patients underwent surgery and even had their stomachs removed, when all they really needed was antibiotics.

The same can be seen with alternative treatments. Thirty years ago, when acupuncture was first introduced to North America, it was considered barbaric quackery. Today, the benefits of acupuncture are well recognized, thanks to advocates of alternative medicine and patients' hands-on experience. The same can also be said about the emergence of energy medicine and the quality-of-life impact it is making on patients with chronic disease.

More than Safe

A growing body of research, especially in Europe, is revealing the many ways in which bioidentical hormones help to improve overall health, with no known harmful side effects. Nearly 200 studies indicate that they are effective in alleviating age-related symptoms with the added benefit of reducing the risk for certain cancers and other diseases. Most recently, Dr. Kent Holtorf's article in *Postgraduate Medicine* quotes 196 articles that show that bioidentical hormones are safer and more effective than synthetic altered hormones. Also, a white paper, extensively researched by the Life Extension Foundation, is very definitive about the benefits of bioidentical hormones compared to synthetic hormones. In plain language, this is not new medicine; it is proven medicine.

Research studies show that bioidentical progesterone can prevent bone loss in patients with a history of osteoporosis. You often hear how estrogen is used to help treat this condition, but it is progesterone that builds bone. So if this applies to you, then you may need to take bioidentical progesterone for the rest of your life, and include weight resistance exercises in your lifestyle.

A French study of 80,000 post-menopausal females found that, over a period of eight years, the risk of breast cancer increased by up to 69 percent in women taking progestins (a synthetic form of progesterone that is not bioidentical). But it decreased by 10 percent among women taking bioidentical progesterone. There are many other studies that mirror these results. When it comes to safety concerns, bioidentical progesterone has been shown to protect against breast cancer in every study.

Its ability to protect against heart disease prompted the president of the American Heart Association to state that a woman who changes her medication from artificial progesterone or medroxyprogesterone acetate (Provera) to natural progesterone would significantly lower her risk of heart disease. Natural progesterone increases HDL cholesterol, the "good" cholesterol that is "cardioprotective," which does not apply to progestins. This is a factor in the increased risk for heart disease, heart attack, and stroke from using the synthetic drug compared to natural progesterone.

A Mayo Clinic study of 176 women compared the quality of life in menopause with the use of bioidentical progesterone. The results indicated significant improvement in issues such as hot flashes, sleep, libido, depression, and anxiety compared to patients taking synthetic progestins.

Synthetic progestins are similar, but not identical, to the hormones produced within the body. Initially developed as contraceptive agents, these drugs are far more potent than natural or bioidentical progesterone, as they can cause an imbalance that leads to devastating side effects. One of the most common progestins is linked to acne, blood clots, weight gain, depression, fluid retention, and some cancers. Few doctors will inform women about these side effects. Many women have blamed themselves when they experience mood swings, bouts of anger, and heightened sensitivity triggered by ingesting this synthetic hormone. These symptoms do not appear when women are given bioidentical progesterone.

More research has dispelled the unwarranted fear that supplementing men with testosterone would lead to prostate cancer. The facts are proving the reverse: it is a lack of testosterone that causes the problem. Testosterone protects against prostate cancer because it helps the immune system to fight it. Weight gain, unrelieved stress, and age have all been proven to cause declining testosterone levels in men. A rapidly expanding collection of research is showing that optimizing testosterone in men also lowers the risk of heart disease, including angina; lowers cholesterol levels; decreases depression; decreases a major cause of heart disease and diabetes; and improves muscle mass, libido, and sexual function.

We're just beginning to realize how much of a role declining testosterone plays in coronary heart disease; it's as much a risk factor as, if not greater than, cholesterol, high blood pressure, or diabetes. From a medical perspective, a testosterone level in the lower-third range with its implications in cardiac disease will significantly affect a man's mortality. The results of one recent study, presented at The Endocrine Society's 91st Annual Meeting in 2009 [newswise.com], concluded that, in middle-aged and older men with low testosterone levels, long-term testosterone replacement therapy significantly improves both liver function and risk factors for cardiovascular disease and diabetes.

This study involved 122 men aged 36 to 69 years, and covered two years of hormone-replacement treatment. Restoring their testosterone to normal levels led to improvements in men diagnosed with "metabolic syndrome" risk factors. Specifically, their weight, waistline measurement, and body mass index (a measure of body fat) continued to decline over the full study period, and 77 percent of those affected no longer had the diagnosis after two years of treatment.

I have seen these results. I know how inserting a pellet of bioidentical testosterone under a man's skin has dramatically improved the quality of his life. Many of my male patients have experienced compelling reversals in their aging symptoms and a substantial improvement in their health.

Europe is far ahead of North America when it comes to studies and ongoing research. The E3N-EPIC cohort study revealed the reduced risk of breast cancer when estrogens are combined with bioidentical progesterone. This benefit comes without the major complications of taking synthetic progestins, which have also been shown to be carcinogenic.

There are more than 20 circulating estrogens in the body with the main players being estriol (E3), estradiol (E2), and estrone (E1). Estrone and estradiol are potent estrogens, and are generally thought to be procarcinogenic when acting alone. Estriol is not carcinogenic. It has the weakest estrogen activity, which is believed to be due to a mixture of pro-estrogenic and anti-estrogenic effects. It binds and activates estrogen receptor beta on breast cells, a receptor that inhibits breast cell proliferation and prevents breast cancer. (Estrone and estradiol bind to estrogen receptor alpha, which promotes breast cell proliferation and can lead to breast cancer development). It is through this mechanism that estriol is believed to confer a protective effect against the development of breast cancer. Adding estriol to estradiol or estrone neutralizes the pro-carcinogenic effects of these powerful estrogens. This is why I will prescribe compounded transdermal creams with a high estriol concentration over estradiol in a 80/20 split (the estradiol-specific stimulation to cells is countered without compromising the beneficial effects on a woman's brain, heart, and bone that is specific to estradiol).

As discussed further in chapter 4, estradiol can be metabolized to either a potent carcinogenic compound, 16-hydroxyesterone, or a non-carcinogenic compound, 2-hydroxyestrone. Post-menopausal women with the highest

16-hydroxyestrone compared to 2-hydroxyestrone were shown to have a risk factor for breast cancer that was 32 times that of the control group (in such women, nutritional measures can be undertaken to reverse this metabolization pattern). Estriol does not convert to the carcinogenic 16-hydroxyestrone, making it a much safer form of estrogen. It also has been demonstrated to cause remission or arrest to breast cancer in 37 percent of post-menopausal women with breast cancer. Estriol has also been proven to improve multiple sclerosis while other estrogens made it worse, which is another indication of the profoundly different effects between the different types of estrogen.

These are just a few examples of the tremendous findings on the safety of bioidentical hormones. Entire books are devoted to the topic and ongoing studies are continuing to add to the research. Bioidentical hormones are the way to go; the studies show that they are very cancer protective, and they help in so many other areas that it's akin to a holistic domino effect.

The Sex Hormones

The three main sex hormones are estrogen and progesterone for women and testosterone for men. However, the sexes do have some overlap; women have smaller requirements for testosterone, just as men have smaller requirements for estrogen. All these hormones diminish as we age. There are more than 50 subsets of hormones but the "big three" are the prime focus because they can cause havoc in our lives when they are out of balance.

Good thyroid functioning is also critical to hormonal balance (see the section below on thyroid malfunction, a very common problem that goes largely undiagnosed). In addition, to give you a good overall picture of hormone health, there are three others to include: DHEA, which forms the basis for the biochemical actions of other hormones (see below); insulin, which is created by the pancreas; and cortisol, which is secreted by the adrenals. The latter two will be discussed in chapters 4 and 5, respectively.

While these hormones are always seen in isolation, they are more like an integrated orchestra, taking cues from one another; if one is off key, the whole orchestra will be out of tune. To add to the dilemma, the hormones that increase as we age (insulin and cortisol) also start to break us down, while the ones that keep us youthful start to diminish.

I believe that, just because the levels of our sex hormones must drop, it doesn't mean that we have to live with this condition. As a practitioner of holistic, functional medicine, I have experienced the compelling results of using bioidentical hormones. I know it is possible to reverse the decline and recapture the hearty, energetic vigor of our youth.

Hormonal fluctuations age us and weaken our quality of life. Slowly and incrementally, we experience symptoms of fatigue, depression, low libido, weight gain, water retention, headaches, mood swings, insomnia, and poor concentration. All of these symptoms may seem overwhelming, and can be devastating. But bioidentical hormones can quite literally change a person's life. Even as a physician, the results are startling, and the rewards have been countless.

I must point out that ingesting bioidentical hormones, such as estrogen and testosterone, is not the preferred option (although it's fine for progesterone). These hormones are metabolized in the body through different pathways; the oral pathway is not a good choice. They can create a lot of clotting factors in the liver and increase the bad cholesterol and fat content that increases the risk of strokes and heart attacks. I always recommend transdermals, such as creams, patches, or under-skin pellets. Almost 90 percent of patients prefer transdermal usage.

You can push the benefits of the good, oral pathway by eating the right foods to enhance your health, especially hardy root vegetables that will be discussed in the next chapter. In addition, always remember that gentle, consistent exercise helps hormones to better metabolize and your body to be more youthfully energetic, strong, and healthy.

Whole-Body Powerhouse

Dehydroepiandrosterone (DHEA) is known as the father of all hormones because it forms the basis for the biochemical actions of other hormones, including testosterone, estrogen, progesterone, and corticosterone. It is mainly secreted through the adrenal cortex (it is the most abundant adrenal steroid hormone) in both men and women; approximately 10 percent is secreted by the ovaries. Small amounts are also produced by adipose tissue, the brain, and in the skin. It is vital for metabolism, energy output, endocrine mechanisms, and reproduction, and has an unusually wide variety of physiological benefits.

I probably put all of my patients on DHEA because of the tremendous associated benefits, which include an overall increase in well-being, mood, sexuality, and energy levels and a decrease in anxiety. However, it is important to monitor DHEA levels through salivary testing during transdermal supplementation because, for example, 50 percent of women will convert it into testosterone. Salivary testing measures only the free DHEA.

Too much testosterone in women can result in facial hair and acne. But if a woman needs testosterone, her body cannot produce it if she is low in DHEA. So I'll put her on DHEA first to determine if she will convert it to testosterone. If not, then I'll supplement with testosterone.

Supplementation with DHEA from early middle age is a key factor in remaining healthy and vitally strong. According to a growing body of research, two of the most fearful, debilitating impairments of old age, Alzheimer's dementia and multi-infarct dementia (the result of numerous mini-strokes), are connected with low DHEA levels.

Studies show that DHEA contributes to the proper growth of brain cells, decreases the formation of blood clots and the stickiness of platelets that can clump to cause heart attacks and strokes, enhances overall immunity, and decreases the symptoms of an enlarged prostate. DHEA helps to reduce menopausal symptoms and regulate hormones; helps to increase muscle mass, builds bone (for osteoporosis prevention), and boosts endurance; lowers LDL cholesterol, stabilizes blood sugar, and reduces age-related increases in insulin levels and insulin resistance; inhibits the conversion of carbohydrates to fats; and inhibits appetite and discourages eating.

DHEA levels peak between 20 and 30 years of age, and then decline until they are approximately 20 percent of peak values by the age of 70. This natural decline coincides with the onset of diseases associated with the aging process. The result has been intense interest in DHEA; there have been thousands of scientific articles published on its metabolic and health properties over the last 50 years. Low levels of this steroid hormone have been associated with many conditions, including rheumatic disease, cardiovascular disease, immune-system disorders, and osteoporosis.

DHEA has been shown to combat adrenal fatigue and support the healthy functioning of the adrenal glands, which control excess cortisol. Since cortisol tends to remain constant or increase with age (and with severe or prolonged stress), whereas DHEA drops dramatically with age or stress, it is obvious that there is a lifelong benefit to maintaining prime levels of DHEA.

I will often use a transdermal application because of its good absorption through the skin. It will enter directly into the cells and this method of delivery will limit the development of sex hormone-binding globulin by the liver which can bind DHEA and other helpful hormones.

Thyroid Traumas

According to my research and nutritional background, in general, one out of four people has a thyroid problem and it is usually undiagnosed. Most traditional doctors rely on blood tests that are ineffective in diagnosing a problem. Practitioners of functional medicine—a holistic approach that engages body, mind, and spirit—know that, in the United States, these acceptable ranges are completely off.

We like to say, when all else fails, look and listen and examine the patient; don't just look at the numbers. Review the lab results to confirm what you're seeing, but in the end talk to the patient to understand how they're feeling; this is a huge failure in traditional medicine. Relying only on test results can cause a patient to suffer needlessly from an undiagnosed condition.

Let's set the scene for this discussion by reviewing the function of the thyroid gland, which is to convert iodine, found in many foods, into two thyroid hormones. These hormones, thyroxine (T4) and triiodothyronine (T3), influence every organ, tissue, and cell in the body through metabolism, heart rate, body weight, body temperature, energy level, and muscle strength.

The thyroid gland is controlled by the pituitary gland, which is controlled by the hypothalamus, an ancient organ within the cerebrum that directs a whole ensemble of hormones. In simplistic terms, the hypothalamus monitors the level of T3 and T4 in the blood; when these levels are suboptimal, it directs the pituitary to send out a thyroid-stimulating hormone (TSH) to the thyroid. This signal stimulates thyroid production of T3 and T4 until blood levels register as "normal," and then it shuts down. T4 represents about 80 percent of the total hormone produced by the thyroid, while T3 represents the remainder.

However, T3 is the much more active hormone (about 300 percent more active) and is responsible for running the metabolic machinery inside all cells. Since T4 is a relatively inactive hormone, to stimulate metabolism in the body it must first be converted to the more active thyroid hormone, T3. Eighty percent of T3 is produced outside the thyroid gland through this conversion in the liver and within the cells of the body.

A nasty blow. Sometimes when you get a head blow early in life, it affects your pituitary, which can drastically impact the secretion of endocrine and growth hormones. During the patient history, I always ask if they have ever had a head blow or concussion that could affect their hormones. The damage from such a traumatic brain injury does not have to be life-threatening. As Dr. Gordon describes in his book, *The Clinical Application of Interventional Endocrinology*, the mechanism of injury can be from: "a minor injury arising from a motor vehicle accident, boxing, martial arts, wrestling, football, skiing, a slip and fall, blunt head trauma, shaken or vibratory pneumatic equipment, sudden drop with sudden stop (amusement park rides), rotation forces, and roller coaster rides."

These types of trauma result in hypopituitarism in 35 to 40 percent of patients where the most common alterations appear to be gonadotropin (estrogen and testosterone) and somatotropin (growth hormone) deficiency, followed by corticotropin (cortisol) and thyrotropin (thyroid) deficiency. This will translate into a myriad of symptoms (see Table 3.1) that are related to the impairment of the brain's ability to regulate these hormones. Treatment must be geared to hormone replacement of demonstrated deficiencies to improve functioning and the quality of life in these survivors of major and minor traumatic brain injuries.

Table 3.1:	Symptoms of Traumatic Brain Injury Syndrome
Excessive sleepiness	Irritability
Inattention	Emotional outbursts
Difficulty concentrating	Disturbed sleep
Impaired memory	Diminished libido
Faulty judgment	Slowed thinking
Depression	Difficulty switching between two tasks

Two thyroid issues. There are two different hypothyroid conditions, both of which often go unrecognized by traditional medical practitioners. Type I hypothyroidism is the complete failure of the thyroid to produce sufficient quantities of thyroid hormone to keep the body running properly; it can be diagnosed with blood tests. This form of hypothyroidism requires ongoing thyroid supplementation, often for the rest of your life. Type II hypothyroidism is a peripheral resistance syndrome where the target cells do not respond properly to the thyroid hormones. This form of hypothyroidism cannot be diagnosed with blood tests, as they will be found to be normal. Due to genetic and environmental factors, this type of hypothyroidism is occurring in epidemic proportions in our population, with some estimates of prevalence as high as 80 percent.

The distinction between the two types of hypothyroidism parallels the distinction between the two types of diabetes. Type I diabetes is the failure of the pancreas gland to produce sufficient insulin to metabolize blood glucose. In Type II diabetes, the body produces sufficient amounts of insulin but the tissues of the body are insensitive to the insulin (insulin resistant), which results in much less efficient metabolism of glucose.

Diagnosing and treating Type I conditions. Type I hypothyroidism is often undiagnosed because a traditional doctor often looks only at the TSH level in the blood and not at the presenting symptoms. If your TSH level is high (around 4 or 5), most doctors will say, "Oh, you're not hypothyroid. Your TSH is in the correct range so your T4 and T3 hormones are being activated." But we have seen many women with levels between 2 and 4 who are hypothyroid, and I'm talking classic Type I hypothyroid with all the symptoms (see Table 3.2).

Table 3.2: Signs and Symptoms of Hypothyroidism			
Symptom	**% of cases**	**Symptom**	**% of cases**
Weakness	99	Constipation	61
Dry skin	97	Weight gain	59
Coarse skin	97	Hair loss	57
Lethargy	91	Pallor of lips	57
Slow speech	91	Dyspnea	55
Edema of eyelids	90	Peripheral edema	55
Sensation of cold	89	Hoarseness	55
Decreased sweating	89	Anorexia	45
Cold skin	83	Nervousness	35
Thick tongue	82	Irregular periods	32
Edema of face	79	Palpitation	31
Coarseness of hair	76	Deafness	30
Pallor of skin	67	Precordial pain	25
Memory impairments	66		

There are two problems with TSH: the lab values are incorrect and they're set too high. In 2002, the American Association of Clinical Endocrinologists recommended the values should be reset between 0.3 and 3, but traditional doctors are still using the older higher range. As I always say, the action's in the middle. We want to see TSH levels that are below 2; around 5 is too high and something is not working right. Doctors who only rely on this test may think that their patients are fine, even though the patient is talking to them and it's evident that they're hypothyroid. Relying on a high TSH will miss up to 80 percent of people with low thyroid.

In addition, most conventional doctors rely on a TSH value that is more reflective of T4 levels and will miss hypothyroid patients that have low T3 levels. Although people can have low T3 due to a dysfunction of the thyroid gland, it is mainly caused by the body's inability to convert T4 to T3.

Table 3.3: Factors That Cause an Inability to Convert T4 to T3			
Nutrient Deficiencies	Medications	Other	Diet
Chromium	Beta Blockers	Aging	Cruciferous Vegetables
Copper	Birth Control Pills	Alcohol	Soy
Iodine	Estrogen	Alcohol	
Iron	Iodinated Contrast Agents	Lipoic Acid	
Selenium	Lithium	Lead	
Zinc	Phenytoin	Lead	
Vitamin A	Steroids	Mercury	
Vitamin B12	Theophylline	Pesticides	
Vitamin B6	Amiodarone	Radiation	
Vitamin B12		Stress	
		Surgery	
		Dieting	
		Hepatic or renal dysfunction	
		Systemic illness	
		Trauma, post-operative state	
		Increased cortisol	

There are several potential causes of this problem, including nutritional deficiencies of iodine, zinc, selenium, and Vitamins A, B6, and B12. Also, a low T3 level can be caused by drugs that block this conversion (e.g., beta blockers, lithium) and drugs that cause T4 to be bound up by proteins in the blood stream (see Table 3.3). This binding up of thyroid hormone occurs because some drugs, such as birth control pills that contain estrogen, increase the amount of thyroxine binding globulin (TBG) that, by its binding effect, decreases the amount of thyroid available for the body to use. TBG helps T4 to get from the thyroid gland to the target organs, but in this bound state it is not metabolically active. This is one reason why I do not use oral estrogen in my therapies; it leads to this binding effect and the resulting hypothyroid symptoms, whereas transdermal preparations do not.

In addition, under physical (particularly due to elevated toxic metals) and emotional stress, the body will convert less T3 from T4 and convert more T4 to reverse T3 (RT3) to conserve energy. The amount of T3 that is converted peripherally can drop by 50 percent with a corresponding increase in RT3 by 50 percent. RT3 can then further inhibit conversion of T4 to T3 by competitive inhibition since the enzyme responsible for both conversions must do double duty. T4 and RT3 compete for the attention of the same enzyme that is involved in the conversion of T4 to T3 and the conversion of RT3 to T2. The result is that more T4 converts to RT3, and the cycle continues (this is known as Wilson's Temperature Syndrome). When the body shunts T4 away from T3, and more toward RT3, the body's cells slow down as RT3 is totally inactive. RT3 is a stereoisomer of T3 and has no biological activity. Dr. Martin Milner of the National College of Naturopathic Medicine describes this situation very well:

"T4 can be compared to a key that has not yet been cut by a locksmith to fit in the lock (the thyroid receptor site). When it is cut properly (as T3), it fits in the lock and opens the door. The RT3 stereoisomer of T3 is a mirror image of the active T3 molecule: a key that is cut differently enough by the locksmith that fits in the lock (receptor site) yet doesn't open the door. When there is an excess of RT3, no thyroid metabolism is stimulated."

The result is that the signs of hypothyroidism begin to recur. Relying on the TSH without obtaining RT3 and T3 levels will reassure a doctor, as TSH will remain normal. But it will leave many patients in distress from the symptoms of hypothyroidism.

Obtaining these levels is also important for quality of life; low levels of T3 and high levels of RT3 will result in an increased risk of death due to congestive heart failure in cardiac patients, and increase the risk of developing the onset of postoperative atrial fibrillation, fibromyalgia, and chronic fatigue syndrome.

The net effect of all these actions is that symptoms of hypothyroidism can still be present even though the TSH is normal. This is the reason why 50 percent of 710 hypothyroid patients stated that they were not satisfied with their treatment, as reported in a quality-of-life survey, the first of its kind, conducted by Mary J. Shomon (thyroid.about.com).

To treat the Type I condition, I prescribe desiccated glandular thyroid products (such as Armour Thyroid, Nature Throid, or Westhroid). These products contain T4 and T3 combinations that make them clinically superior to synthetic versions (such as Synthroid or Levothroid) that contain only T4 because the body is able to convert the desiccated hormone to the active hormone more efficiently. This is in part due to other active ingredients present in the glandular product including calcitonin, selenium, and small amounts of thyroid hormones, T2 and T1. The decades-old argument by conventional medicine against the use of desiccated thyroid, that it is not consistent from dose to dose, does not hold up in research studies nor does it hold up in my experience.

The treatment for all patients should be individualized since, as with any hormone therapy, there is no such thing as a "one size fits all" treatment. Everyone is different; some will be helped tremendously with Armour Thyroid but some will not. It can depend on how far gone the thyroid is.

Let's say that you have an autoimmune problem that has gone unrecognized for years and has caused a lot of damage (the average time is seven years before traditional medicine picks up on this type of an autoimmune problem). In that time, your thyroid can be partially or completely destroyed, your body has built up antibodies against it, and it may never completely regain its optimal functioning state. You have to be on thyroid medication for the rest of your life. However, there are many cases where you can actually stop the autoimmunity condition in time and then, through good nutrition and exercise, it's possible to restore the effective thyroid functions.

Treating Type II hypothyroidism. The Type II condition is found in epidemic levels in today's modern society, particularly among women, and it is not revealed through standard blood tests. A woman, for example, can have a normal blood test result and yet she'll say, "Doctor, I cannot lose weight, my hands and feet feel cold, I have constipation, I'm losing hair, I have a problem with my aches and pains, and I cannot think." If you talk to her, you know that she's hypothyroid; however, if you look at the lab readings, she presents as normal. This is thyroid resistance; for some reason, the cells' receptors are not recognizing thyroid hormones as they should.

There could be many reasons for this condition. It is found in individuals with genetic anomalies, with long-standing fibromyalgia or chronic fatigue syndrome, in people taking excessive calcium, extreme caloric restriction, pregnancy, emotional stress, and in adrenal fatigue. Certain nutritional deficiencies can also be factors; they include iodine, selenium, zinc, Vitamin C, Vitamin B, and Vitamin A. All of these are useful in trying to shock the cells into recognizing circulating thyroid hormones.

These nutritional deficiencies may be why the Type II problem occurred, but a poor diet, including too many refined carbohydrates, food additives, and toxins, is a major cause of this condition. The classic cause is an imbalance in a woman's hormones that creates an estrogen-dominant condition found in perimenopause and menopause. This can also interfere with her cells' ability to recognize the T3 and T4 thyroid hormones, and why women complain that they cannot lose weight during this transition despite being on exercise and diet programs.

The Type II condition can be reversed with a commitment to diet and lifestyle changes along with nutraceutical supplements, detoxification of the body, and a therapeutic trial of sustained release T3 hormone to overcome the resistance and reverse the signs of hypothyroidism. Sustained release T3 is preferable as the short half-life of immediate release T3 (0.75 days), such as Cytomel, is more likely to result in side effects. These side effects include, but are not limited to, rapid heart rate, irregular pulse, anxiety, nervousness, agitation, irritability, sweating, headaches, increased bowel motility, and menstrual irregularities. Also, angina, congestive heart failure, and atrial fibrillation can be aggravated or induced by excessive doses of T3.

Correcting Thyroid Imbalance

Some symptoms of aging can show up as early as the mid-twenties. Impotence, pre-menstrual syndrome, fatigue, and similar ailments are indicators that something is out of balance, and will continue to remain unbalanced until it completely saps your vitality in later years. By the time Wanda Lee (I have changed the names of patients throughout this book to protect their privacy) came to me at the age of 30, she was struggling with a thyroid problem that had been in existence for a long time, and her symptoms were only increasing.

Her story is an example of the dramatic results that can come from correctly diagnosing and treating a thyroid imbalance with bioidentical hormones. Wanda had seen many doctors, including endocrinologists, without success. This patient looked and felt like a very unhappy young woman. She had stopped menstruating. "I had not had a period for eleven months," Wanda recalls. She was also gaining weight. Depressed and lethargic, she complained of various aches and pains, and constipation. These are classic symptoms of hypothyroidism.

While I recognized the symptoms, diagnosing thyroid conditions is not clear cut and one reason why so many doctors do not diagnose the problem correctly. You have to figure it out based on talking with the patient; conducting follow-up tests; and relying on the hindsight of experience by looking for red flags such as feeling cold, gaining weight, experiencing aches and pains, losing hair, and the other classic symptoms of hypothyroidism.

In Wanda's case, her test results indicated that her thyroid was functioning in the normal range (which I've mentioned is set too high for many people). One problem in many clinical settings is that no one listens to the patient; they just look at the numbers. Wanda knew that something wasn't functioning right; she had spent two years searching for answers. So our treatment was to not just test the TSH range but also tyrosine kinase, which is important in the production of thyroid hormones.

Wanda had been taking a synthetic medication so I prescribed Armour Thyroid, at a dosage specific to her condition, to be taken three to four times a day. The results with this bioidentical hormone were rather dramatic. Her natural enthusiasm came back in six months; she started to have more energy and lose weight, and her periods began returning. "With bioidentical hormone therapy, I am now happier, calmer, more energetic, and sleeping better than I have in years," she says.

As her doctor, I can't believe that she is the same person; she's now very active and the zest for life that was absent from my first visit with her returned. Wanda's life has turned around so much that she wants to help other people who are experiencing what she went through. She's so enthusiastic about our approach that she always stops by and asks, "Do you have a job for me yet?"

Weary Women

The traditional medical community believes that women should limit prolonged use of hormone drugs. They should only long take it enough to obtain relief from menopausal symptoms and then no more. But ample research shows that women will safety benefit from individualized doses of natural estrogens and progesterone over their lifetime, as it will support the quality of their days and protect against bone loss, certain cancers, and other debilitating diseases.

Each year, millions of women are prescribed antidepressants for symptoms such as depression, mood dysfunctions, and insomnia when their bodies are in dire need of estrogen. A study in the *Journal of Reproductive Medicine* reported a statistical analysis of depressed women in psychiatric hospitals. Results indicated that 41 percent were admitted either the day before or on the first day of their menses.

When their estrogen levels dip, such as during natural fluctuations in their monthly cycle or at any stage of life, many women have said that they felt depressed, flat, uninspired, or hopeless. These feelings are a direct result of estrogen deficiency. The restorative power of bioidentical estrogen offers hope for many women suffering unnecessarily.

Progesterone is also the natural Prozac for women; it's the calming hormone.

In most cases, along with bioidentical estrogen I might also use natural progesterone because of its complementary benefits. Progesterone has anti-proliferative effects on breast tissue that is antagonistic to the proliferative effects of estrogen. It up-regulates the gene that causes cancer cells to die (a process known as apoptosis). As a result, unlike synthetic progestins, multiple studies show that progesterone is not associated with an increase in breast cancer. Progesterone is also the natural Prozac for women; it's the calming hormone. Produced by the ovaries and the adrenal glands in women, and in smaller amounts in the testes and the adrenal glands in men, it plays an important role in brain function.

Low levels of progesterone can cause increased feelings of anxiety, irritability, and anger. When progesterone is metabolized, it binds with gamma amino butyric acid (GABA) receptors in the brain. GABA acts as a neurotransmitter (a chemical transmitter of information between nerve cells) and has a calming effect on the brain. Bioidentical progesterone helps to support this process, suppresses mood swings, and promotes a whole-body calmness.

Progesterone is the body's oldest steroid hormone; it is about 500 million years old on the evolutionary scale. All vertebrates produce progesterone, although only in higher vertebrates is this hormone instrumental in the reproductive cycle. The difference between the synthetic form, such as medroxyprogesterone, and natural, bioidentical progesterone is that the former can actually lower a patient's natural production of progesterone.

Some women who are prescribed an oral, synthetic progesterone to combat premenstrual syndrome (PMS), irregular menses, or estrogen dominance will report side effects such as headaches, mood swings, or fluid retention. But in its natural micronized form, bioidentical progesterone acts as a diuretic; women who take it may have to use the bathroom more frequently but they are spared the bloating and weight gain of synthetic progestin. These women also report their mood swings will often diminish, and many who suffer from migraines as part of PMS get relief from this as well.

So a 34-year-old woman, for example, who is estrogen dominant (she has more estrogen in proportion to the progesterone in her body) will likely be unable to sleep and will feel anxious; she may have heart palpitations and is probably depressed. That woman needs progesterone.

Estrogen dominance is the result of being overweight, under excessive stress, or due to the absorption of artificial estrogens (zenoestrogens, which will be discussed in chapter 8) from the environment. Symptoms such as breast tenderness, water retention, mood swings, irritability, foggy thinking, depression, food cravings, weight gain, anxiety, and night sweats are lessened with bioidentical progesterone. Progesterone's calming effect is complemented by its role in the production and regulation of other hormones such as cortisol, testosterone, and estrogen, and it can also help to balance these hormones.

Perils of perimenopause. Before a woman reaches the menopausal stage, which is clinically defined as no periods for at least 12 months, they will go through a perimenopausal phase with symptoms lasting five to ten years before menopause hits. These women can be in their mid- to late thirties or even younger, due to exposure to environmental and artificial estrogens, including birth control pills. They need to be treated because they can suffer greatly. Just because a woman is 38, it doesn't mean, "No, doctor, don't treat her until she's menopausal," because the quality of her life is already going down; she can suffer for ten years and her self-confidence can nosedive until she's unrecognizable to her family and friends.

She's beginning to lose progesterone while estrogen is still being created by the ovaries. These women often come to me because they cannot sleep. If they cannot sleep, they cannot think or function, and that stresses their adrenal glands; they can gain 10 pounds just from the inability to sleep, which stresses their adrenal glands even further. In addition, perimenopausal women who are low in progesterone (estrogen dominant) cannot lose weight no matter how much they exercise. But once the correct balance is achieved between estrogen, progesterone, and testosterone, this goes away and they start losing weight more easily, even without exercising, because we've balanced their hormones.

Menopause madness. When a woman begins to experience a number of unpleasant symptoms during her menopausal period, the person she once knew, the vibrant person who wasn't afraid to go to Europe by herself, explore new places, or hike into the woods, begins to disappear. She's weaker, her bones are thinner, she's depressed, and has lost the enthusiasm of her youth. Now she's become this person who's afraid to do anything because her body is no longer reliable; she has lost confidence in her body.

As a woman goes fully into menopause and her ovaries shut down, her estrogen levels slowly diminish. Her libido can weaken or vanish at this time because her testosterone is dipping. So not only does she lose her sex drive, intercourse is now painful because of vaginal dryness.

We know that 87 percent of women with a hormonal imbalance have genitourinary symptoms. With bioidentical hormone therapy, 50 percent of these women will have relief from their symptoms by using a skin patch, gel or pills, but 95 percent will get relief with intravaginal hormone replacement therapy. The effectiveness of vaginal delivery of hormones, including estriol, estrone, progesterone, and testosterone, has been well established in the literature. These intravaginal hormones are absorbed systemically and are biologically active to relieve the symptoms of menopause. The advantage is that it bypasses the liver; vaginal hormone replacement therapy does not affect clotting factors, which may increase the risk of clot formation. In addition, there are no adverse effects to the lipid profiles (increase of bad cholesterol or triglycerides) or blood pressure.

I will supplement with intravaginal, bioidentical estrogen, particularly estriol, to correct vaginal dryness. Studies have demonstrated that the use of this low-potency estrogen will also increase bone density (unlike oral estriol) without the increased risk of endometrial hyperplasia or uterine cancer and breast cancer. Depending on the results of a saliva or 24-hour urinary hormone study, I may identify that my patient will benefit from a combination of estrogen, progesterone, and testosterone, taken intravaginally as well as in topical form.

For women in menopause, the flexibility of bioidentical hormones can bring forth quite dramatic results. Weight gain, aches and pains, hair loss, and the inability to sleep are all alleviated. The inability to sleep is a common presenting symptom and bioidentical progesterone will help, especially in cases of not being able to fall asleep and stay asleep. Many women can readily fall asleep but invariably wake up within a two- to four-hour window. However, progesterone taken orally metabolizes well, and it triggers receptors in the brain that allow these women to sleep throughout the night.

During the day, the use of progesterone in tandem with estrogen helps with alertness and concentration, which can be a challenge as hormones diminish with age. For women with systemic side effects from oral progesterone, such as bloating, sleepiness, or persistent hot flashes, intravaginal progesterone has proven beneficial without increasing the risk of breast cancer. In fact, intravaginal administration of progesterone is preferred in patients with cardiovascular or liver disease, and decreases the metabolic burden on the liver.

Hot flashes and night sweats add to the sleep challenge. Nighttime becomes a constant torment; if they can fall asleep, these women wake up two hours later, or they cannot get to sleep and then wake up frequently through the night. So it becomes a quality-of-life issue. Fully 80 percent of my patients have an issue with sleep. The collective disruption of sleep deprivation and hormonal dips results in a lack of concentration, mood swings, and emotional outbursts. A woman's quality of life declines greatly.

Yet most of these things improve or disappear altogether with bioidentical hormone supplementation, as well as some diet and lifestyle changes. Once a woman has experienced the positive difference in her life, she understandably doesn't want to go back.

With menopausal women, because of the loss of estrogen and progesterone, their skin also starts aging very rapidly. Declining estrogen has been connected with a loss of collagen and elastin in the skin; this is why you get sagging as part of aging. I've seen women in the emergency room who are around 70 years old and their skin easily tears from a fall; that's in part due to a loss of estrogen. Because estrogen helps to preserve the skin's infrastructure, bioidentical

It lifts depression; grows bone and muscle; improves vaginal dryness; and greatly increases libido.

estrogen cream can help cosmetically. Adding exercise, a good diet without sugar, stress reduction, and no smoking will add to your lifelong youthful appearance.

A little known benefit, particularly for athletic women, is that estrogen replacement treatment reverses the loss of lung surface area and repairs the lost and damaged alveoli (the gas exchange area of the lungs) that occurs with normal aging. Menopause further accelerates the loss of lung surface area. Hormone replacement therapy maximizes your lungs' ability to absorb oxygen and get rid of carbon dioxide as you get older. This is important for non-smoking women who developed emphysema but it will also help you with daily routine activities. You will be better able to handle walking up and down store aisles or working in your garden for extended periods. In addition, it will combat the "aging" of your speaking and singing voice.

Finally, bioidentical, non-oral (intravaginal, topical, or pellet implants) testosterone has also significantly improved menopausal symptoms. Testosterone clears up the mental fog of menopause, which helps with concentration and focus. It lifts depression; grows bone and muscle; improves vaginal dryness; and greatly increases libido. It balances the action of estrogen by preventing proliferation of breast tissue (it has a pro-apototic effect, which means that it increases cancer cell death at normal body concentration levels found pre-menopausally), decreases estrogen receptor alpha, and prevents the stimulation of breast tissue from estrogen or progestin therapy. It has been demonstrated clinically to be so breast protective that it has been used to treat patients with advanced breast cancer, with implantation (testosterone pellets underneath the skin) used as part of endocrine therapy in breast cancer survivors.

In women who do not want to be bothered with applying testosterone intravaginally or onto the skin daily, testosterone pellet implantation is a great option. This method of testosterone delivery requires a very simple 15-minute procedure to place a testosterone pellet the size of a rice kernel in the subcutaneous tissue of the upper buttock. The advantage is that a steady stream of testosterone is released as needed, over a four- to six-month period, with complete eradication of menopausal symptoms. With the appropriate indications, testosterone implantation is a godsend to their menopausal symptoms and I find that, once experienced, these women prefer this method of delivery.

Grumpy Older Men

On the whole, nature has been fortunate to men: they don't have as many hormones to worry about, don't have to give birth to babies, and don't have menstrual cycles. However, they still go through their own version of menopause, called andropause, and it's strictly related to their testosterone levels.

Research indicates that men's testosterone peaks at around age 21, and then incrementally diminishes at a rate of one to two percent rate per year. So by the time he's in his sixties, a man's testosterone level is a key concern. Many men will concentrate below the belt on issues such as erection problems and libido. But those symptoms usually happen very late in the game. A variety of hormonal changes are happening before then, with many similar symptoms to a woman's change of life: hot flashes, night sweats, anxiety, trouble with concentration, mood swings, and so forth. The result is what I call the "grumpy older men syndrome."

Men become depressed, anxious, irritable, fatigued, and constipated, with very low libido and difficulty with erections. They can experience aches and pains, a rapid heart rate, and other cardiac problems. And then, of course, men have urinary problems (such as "hesitancy"). Benign prostatic hypertrophy, an enlarged prostate gland, triggers the inability to urinate completely. It is an increasingly common problem as men age.

For men taking long-term, bioidentical testosterone replacement, the rate of this uncomfortable condition is far below that of untreated men. For many of the happy wives of the treated men, the phrase "the South will rise again" has new meaning. The combination of all these issues can be debilitating, affecting not just their own lives but those of their family. When it comes to the symptoms of aging, there's a lot of overlap between how badly women feel and how men struggle. The big difference, however, is that men lose testosterone over 30 years; women lose all their sex hormones within five years. Women's symptoms are hyper-acute, while men's symptoms are more insidious; he knows that something's wrong but can't put his finger on it. So he thinks, "Oh, I've lost my step because I'm getting older." He's not really aware of the slow-and-steady decline in optimal functioning.

With age, the amount of active testosterone in a man's blood decreases. Left behind is a higher proportion of estrogen; from a testosterone to estrogen ratio of 50:1 in a young man, he now has a ratio of between 10:1 and 20:1; so that a 50-year-old man can have more estrogen than a 50-year-old woman. This rising proportion of estrogen increases clotting factors and narrowing of the coronary arteries, leading to an escalating risk of heart attacks (it has the opposite effect in women) and strokes.

On the flip side, the decreasing proportion of testosterone leads to more insulin resistance, as its antagonistic properties to the stress hormones adrenalin and cortisol are now diminishing. In addition, because testosterone is a potent vasodilator due to its stimulation of nitric oxide, its increasing loss leads to gradual reduction in blood flow throughout the body, including the organs that need it most: the brain, heart, and penis. The result is the weight gain, particularly around the belly, increased cholesterol and triglycerides, impotence, high blood pressure, and a very threatened heart. In fact, a low testosterone level is a greater independent risk factor for coronary artery disease than a man's family history, total cholesterol, or smoking habit.

Most of a man's testosterone is bound to other proteins and not readily usable. It is the free testosterone, representing two to three percent of total testosterone, which is unbound and therefore bioactive (it creates activity in all cells where testosterone has a role including the brain, heart, muscle, bone, and gonads). Although men need some estrogen, like women need some testosterone, the effect is all in the balance. With too much estrogen, men double their risk of stroke and increase their risk of coronary artery disease. Too little estrogen predisposes men to osteoporosis and bone fracture.

This is why it is important to check free testosterone and estradiol blood levels in routine lab tests. But it is rarely done in conventional medicine. The implications are profound. A recent study of 3014 men aged 69 to 80 years, who were followed for up to 4.5 years, makes it clear: men with low testosterone had 65 percent greater all-cause mortality, while men with low estradiol suffered 54 percent more deaths. Men who were low in both estradiol and testosterone had a 96 percent increase in mortality; they were almost twice as likely to die compared to men in the optimal ranges.

Too much estrogen in men can arise from a variety of factors. These include increasing aromatase with age and weight gain (this enzyme converts testosterone to estrogen and is found in fat cells), a decreasing effectiveness of the liver (which metabolizes estrogen) due to prescription drug and alcohol use, and zinc deficiency (zinc inhibits levels of aromatase).

Men can get caught in a "wheel of misfortune" cycle where more estrogen is made by aromatase due to increasing weight gain as a result of low testosterone levels. The result is a depletion of more vital testosterone while increasing estradiol to unsafe ranges. In addition, estrogen increases the production of sex hormone-binding globulin (SHBG) that binds testosterone, leading to less bioactive free testosterone availability, and the downward cycle continues.

Interrupting this cycle with a treatment regime of testosterone replacement, vitamin and mineral supplementation, liver detoxification, and lifestyle changes is critically important for the mature man's health and vitality as he ages. Testosterone replacement can be in the form of creams, patches, sublingual pellets, injections, or pellet implantation. Pellet implantation is similar to the procedure for women but with significantly more pellets implanted. Before starting the treatment, and at periodic intervals during treatment, a physical exam and blood tests should be performed. Blood tests should include a total or free Prostate-Specific Antigen (PSA) test or the newly approved human aspartyl (asparaginyl) beta-hydroxylase (HAAH) prostate cancer test.

Have you ever wonder what happened to your libido when you started your statin drug to lower your cholesterol? While effectively reducing your cholesterol levels, it also decreases your testosterone. Cholesterol is the source of all sex hormones, including testosterone, estrogen, and DHEA. Reducing cholesterol to the low levels now recommended by the American Heart Association for prevention, or for high-risk patients, will also trigger a reduction in coenzyme Q-10, essential fatty acids, and Vitamin D levels. This will result in increased inflammation, leading to increased risk of heart disease and cancer and higher mortality. To prevent sexual dysfunction and other issues arising from taking these drugs, it is better to institute healthier lifestyle changes including exercise, stress reduction, and antioxidant supplementation.

When I insert a pellet of bioidentical testosterone under an older man's skin, his life is transformed; he becomes a different person. The improvement is so acute that he cannot live without his bioidentical hormone therapy because he now remembers what he felt like when he was young. The simple addition of testosterone helps him to regain the potent, vibrant strength of his youth.

As an example, one patient loved athletics but at the age of 65 was losing muscle strength and the energy to maintain his level of exercise. Now on bioidentical testosterone, he is out-lifting his son in weights. He regained the testosterone needed to achieve this, and is gaining body mass where he never had it before. This man is so enthusiastic about the difference in his life that he emailed photos to show that he could bench press more than his son.

Bioidentical Hormones are Affordable

The benefits of bioidentical hormones have been in the spotlight due to the endorsement of some celebrities, but it is truly an affordable wellness approach. You can expect your costs to be about $100 to $150 per month for treatment, depending on your age and symptoms. Some insurance companies may even cover the costs.

When I first see a patient, I usually give the hormones separately because I want him or her to feel better quickly. As soon as I see an improvement, I'll combine the hormones into a compound treatment to make it more cost effective.

In addition, my holistic treatment includes education about a health-enhancing diet and dynamic lifestyle choices to bring about permanent results. Many patients will spend hundreds of dollars per month on quick, weight loss diets and then regain the weight, or more, after they drop out of the program. So this investment is truly cost effective.

In summary, this chapter represents the tip of the iceberg when it comes to the complex and fascinating world of hormones. Before the ink dries on these pages, there will be new research and knowledge to benefit our lives, and that can only enhance the health and longevity of maturing men and women.

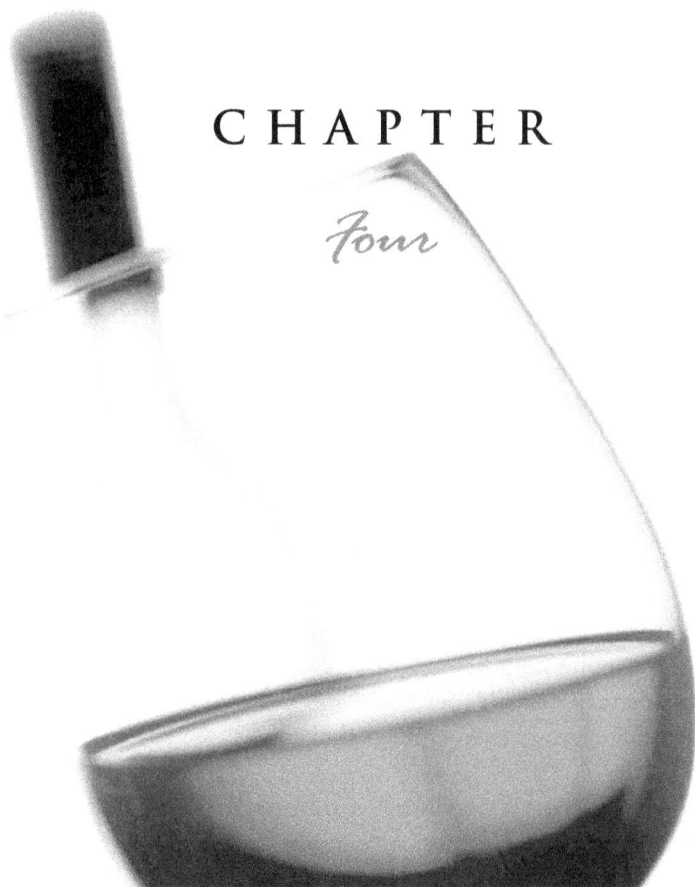

CHAPTER

Four

CHAPTER FOUR

Food For Thought

*"Everyone has a doctor in him or her; we just have
to help it in its work. The natural healing force within
each one of us is the greatest force in getting well. Our food
should be our medicine. Our medicine should be our food."*

Hippocrates

Integrative medicine is about combining alternative, complementary, and conventional therapies to take advantage of the strengths of each while offsetting their weaknesses. Conventional medicine provides a good, scientific understanding of how food affects everything from your moods to the balance of your hormones and your avoidance of diseases. The impact of diet grows even more critical as you age.

Combined with alternative medicine's guidance on eating holistically, this knowledge will help to enhance your health and prevent disease. Your body becomes less tolerant of imbalance on all levels with every age-related milestone. If you wish to remain thoroughly and vigorously in your prime, regardless of your age, strategically effective nutrition is of prime importance.

Quantities of research now highlight the kind of diet that will protect your strength and ensure a robust, healthy future. Certain nutraceutical supplements and power foods are proving to offer specific health benefits.

However, I do not recommend the latest fads in dieting and media-hyped "wonder foods." I must also warn you that I'm not talking about the standard, North American diet because that's what has made so many of us sick.

The power and necessity of food goes far beyond sustaining life. Food affects all areas of your life, including your energy, stamina, digestion, complexion, ability to sleep and handle stress, and desire for sex. Good nutrition forms the building blocks of wellness on which you add nutritional supplements and bioidentical hormone therapy.

More simply, what you put in your mouth will affect your overall happiness for life.

Avoiding the Carb Rush

The high-and-crash that comes with eating too many "bad" carbohydrates is terribly stressful on your body. It sets off a cascade of events that will prematurely age all of your physiological processes. It is a forum for disease, and it has no place in your life if you wish to remain zestfully energetic and healthy.

Carbohydrates are essential; they are your energy batteries. Almost all carbohydrates are converted into glucose, the fuel that drives your body. The major sources include plant foods and are classified as either complex or simple carbohydrates.

Complex carbohydrates are starches that consist of many sugar molecules; they include whole grains, legumes, vegetables, and some fruits. These are processed slowly in the digestive system, which is key: the longer timeframe for complex carbohydrates to be broken down into glucose and other nutrients for the bloodstream creates a longer acting, better-burning fuel for maximum health.

Simple carbohydrates, on the other hand, consist of a few sugar molecules and are burned quickly by the body. Modern processing, such as stripping the fiber from grains and removing the pulp from fruit juices, are examples of turning a good, complex carbohydrate into a simple carbohydrate.

These sugary and refined foods have become the staples of the North American diet. We each consume 158 pounds of sugar a year in this diet. They result in a quick start-and-stop effect that fills you with a sugar high; the large and rapid rise in your blood-sugar level causes your pancreas to expel massive amounts of insulin to metabolize all of the extra sugar, which overshoots the target and results in a low blood-sugar level. Then you crash. Eventually, your blood glucose stabilizes until you consume the next refined food. Then the high-and-crash effect repeats itself.

All simple carbohydrates break down into simple sugars. The glycemic index is a measure of this reaction. A high-glycemic food produces very high blood-sugar level. Eating a typical large, white-bread bagel is like eating a spoonful of sugar. It has the same effect on your body. The problem is that all the sugar in a typical North American diet can't be metabolized. At some point, you have so much circulating in your body that it has to be turned into fat, and so you pack on additional weight.

Another dilemma in eating a lot of these sugary foods is that you're playing havoc with your hormones, especially insulin. Over time, the high-and-crash effect leads to insulin resistance. Fat cells will take any calorie you give it, no matter how many. Over time, your cells' insulin receptors begin to diminish.

An average person has about 20,000 insulin receptors per cell, but overweight people have maybe 4000 to 5000 insulin receptors per cell. So all that sugar from overeating is in the bloodstream, and all this insulin is trying to bring the sugar into each cell and metabolize it, but there are now fewer channels in which to do it. The result is a bottleneck; you have elevated levels of sugar and insulin in your blood, which causes your whole body to become inflamed; all the free radicals released in the process are damaging your body.

These include substances called advanced glycation end products (AGEs) and advanced lipoxidation end products (ALEs), which are formed from sugar at a constant but slow rate in a normal body.

AGEs and ALEs bind to the surface of cells, resulting in an avalanche of destructive free radicals and inflammation. They are formed when sugars bind with proteins, amino acids, or fats in the body in a process called glycation. It is believed that AGEs and ALEs are responsible for many kinds of dysfunction in diabetics, including tissue damage found in vascular disease, kidney failure, eye damage, and immune dysfunction. However, AGEs and ALEs develop and will accumulate with age even in non-diabetics. Even though their formation is markedly accelerated with the increased availability of glucose, the effect is the same.

AGEs and ALEs age you quickly, as they cause sagging skin and wrinkles, cataracts, and Alzheimer's disease. They produce cross-linkages that create inflexibility in your arteries, heart, and lungs, which can lead to atherosclerosis and heart failure. Although the glycation process cannot be completely prevented, it can be slowed by reducing your sugar intake. The aging damage from protein and lipid glycation can

Blood sugar must be regulated very tightly and your diet is the blood-sugar machine.

also be reduced by taking Vitamin B6 vitamers, pyridoxamine and pyridoxal-5'-phosphate (different chemical forms of Vitamin B6 with the most anti-glycation activity).

Blood sugar must be regulated very tightly and your diet is the blood-sugar machine. If you choose a whole-grain bagel, the digestion process is more complex. It takes longer to chew and swallow; you tend to eat less; you metabolize it more slowly; the spike of insulin is not as high; and your energy is sustained for a longer period of time.

With a common, on-the-run breakfast, after you have hastily gobbled down your white-bread bagel and sugar-laden coffee, you will have a big insulin / high glycemic / blood-sugar rush. You'll feel good for a little while, but it will be short lived. The high-blood sugar produces serotonin, which is a good mood neurotransmitter to the brain, but after the sugar high and the insulin kicks out, you crash.

Your blood sugar drops; you feel irritable, lethargic, absent-minded, and weak by noon. The brain starts to nag at you, "Oh-oh, we're low in blood sugar, we need a hit," so you grab a snack and the high/low-blood sugar cycle starts all over again. That sugar-induced, poor-eating cycle ultimately leads to insulin resistance. Eventually, your cells become saturated and the cells' healthy insulin receptors diminish.

Curbing the Crash with Protein And Fat

To block that insulin response and reduce highs and lows, include a protein and some essential fatty acid in your fast food meal. This pairing will help to block that high-glycemic response and offset the potential insulin resistance in that meal.

It will lessen the damage. It can be as simple as adding a small amount of cheese or fish (especially salmon), or a few nuts. The high glycemic index of a potato can be blunted by adding protein, especially a complex carbohydrate such as beans or legumes, and a handful of walnuts or almonds. The combination of the trio is key.

Although fruits have a somewhat high glycemic index, the fiber creates a slower release so that you don't get the high-sugar surge that would come from eating a white bread bagel. To block the effects of high-glycemic-index foods, you have to somehow reduce insulin resistance. That's why it is recommended that we eat five to nine portions of fruits and vegetables per day.

Exercise plays another huge role in improving insulin resistance. Add exercise to your day and you can boost the insulin receptors of your cells to about 25,000. This means that you're able to transport and metabolize glucose more efficiently in the cell, which leads to more energy during exercise and throughout your work day. For more information about this topic, see chapter 6.

Diet Differences

Our North American diet is killing us. The carbohydrate crash I just described is one unhealthy aspect. Research leaves no doubt that our meat-centered diet and highly refined meals are contributing toward many common age-related and degenerative illnesses. Every bit of effort that you can make to get off the Western diet wagon will reap ample rewards: greater resistance to disease, superior longevity, and a much higher quality of life.

The Blue Zones by Dan Buettner is a study of cultures with the highest percentage of people living into their nineties and beyond. These people have several important physical, mental, and social traits in common. With regard to food, most of them favor a plant-based, whole-foods diet, and many are outright vegetarians.

Buettner depicts a study of members of the Seventh Day Adventist Church; this group of people in California commonly lives into their second century. From 1974 to 1988, the "Adventist Health Study-1" investigated nearly 34,000 church members over the age of 25.

In addition to a wholesome lifestyle (which I will discuss in greater detail in the coming chapters), approximately half of them were vegetarians or rarely ate meat. Because of his lifestyle, 30-year-old Adventist male will live 7.3 years longer than his California counterpart; and if he's vegetarian, he will add another 2.2 years to this. His female counterpart will live 4.4 years longer than the average; as a vegetarian, she will add another 1.7 years to her lifespan. Not eating meat is clearly extending their lives.

In addition, non-vegetarian Adventists were found to have about twice the risk of heart disease, and a 50 to 65 percent increased risk of colon, bladder, and ovarian cancer, compared to their vegetarian brethren. However, even for the carnivores, the study indicated that eating more legumes, such as peas and beans, offered a 30 to 40 percent reduction in colon cancer. In addition, eating the unsaturated fat in nuts, at least five times a week, cut the risk for heart disease in half, regardless of meat consumption.

Epidemiologists know that consuming fruits, vegetables, and whole grains seems to be protective for a wide variety of cancers. Studies are pointing to nuts' effect on lowering blood cholesterol. This means that a low-meat, plant-based diet is your ticket to long years of high-quality health.

Another book, *The China Study*, details the connection between nutrition and heart disease, diabetes, and cancer. The book's title refers to the China Project, a survey of death rates for more than 2400 counties and 880 million (roughly 96 percent) Chinese people, conducted jointly by Cornell University, Oxford University, and the Chinese Academy of Preventive Medicine over the course of 20 years.

This extremely detailed study concluded that eating a whole-food, plant-based diet and avoiding beef, poultry, and milk helped to minimize or even reverse the development of chronic disease.

Authors T. Colin Campbell, Ph.D., a professor of Nutritional Biochemistry at Cornell University, and his son, Thomas Campbell, conclude that diets high in animal protein (including casein in cow's milk) are strongly linked to such illnesses as cancer of the breast, prostate, and large bowel, diabetes, coronary heart disease, autoimmune diseases, osteoporosis, degenerative brain disease, and macular degeneration, as well as obesity.

If you want a cleansing diet, we know that plant-based foods are best. I have seen studies that indicate we can reverse atherosclerosis (where the arteries are narrowed because the walls have a build-up of fatty materials such as cholesterol) and heart disease by adopting a plant-based diet. A major tenet of traditional medicine was that, once you have atherosclerosis in your coronary arteries, you have it for life. All you can do is have an angioplasty to mechanically widen the blocked artery or a bypass operation. Now we know that it can be reversed.

However, only an entirely plant-based, meat-free diet will reverse this condition. Of course, the problem is that too many people are used to the "standard American diet," and if they have this condition, such a diet will result in severe impairment of their functioning, and even death.

Regaining, or protecting, health requires the willingness to adopt a better-quality lifestyle. As we progress into the 21st century, our main threat is food. We are all exposed to what I call a toxic food environment. From the fast-food restaurants on every corner of our cities to the television and print advertisements, we are constantly bombarded with depictions of mouth-watering, high-fat foods along with desserts, candy, sugary cereals, and soft drinks all clothed within an environment of fostering good family values and good nutrition. This Trojan horse has resulted in an avalanche of the diseases of advanced society in all its abundance: heart attacks, diabetes, high blood pressure, and strokes.

Back in the primitive, hunter-gatherer societies of our ancient history, we were much healthier because we ate to live; now we live to eat. We're eating excessive food and poor-quality food. The sum of all these unhealthy combinations of calories is chronic inflammation throughout the body.

The Weighty Question

The term "inflammaging" depicts how aging is accompanied by a low-grade, chronic, systemic inflammatory response. It was coined by Claudio Franceschi, a professor of the Department of Experimental Pathology, University of Bologna, Italy. Studies clearly show this inflammatory response is common to most age-associated diseases. So combating inflammation is primary to preserving a healthy, dynamic vitality in the prime of your life.

An inflamed body is an unhealthy body, no matter what the cause. But there is a proven link between obesity and inflammation. Cellular stress from excess weight can contribute to chronic inflammation. The added risk of insulin resistance is a precursor to diabetes and other metabolic disorders.

Regardless of the original cause of the obesity, an overweight person is struggling with more than girth and pounds. Inflammation is the body's normal response to injury; it typically promotes healing. But when fat-storing cells, or adipocytes, become enlarged with fat, they produce pro-inflammatory stimuli such as free fatty acids.

These stimuli activate immune cells residing within the tissues, which in turn release pro-inflammatory cytokines, which are messenger chemicals that link cells together. An inflammatory cascade grows, slowly and tragically, into an ongoing overreaction to the obese condition.

Fat cells are not just reservoirs of excess calories. They are living, breathing organs. They create inflammatory markers that go into your brain, crossing the blood-brain barrier and lowering your levels of serotonin and dopamine, bringing down your mood, and impairing your cognitive functioning.

A similar inflammation process is associated with many neurodegenerative diseases. It is implicated in the cognitive and behavioral impairments that are seen in aging. It's all part of the same inflammation cascade. Getting that inflammation under control is critical to your constitution, and staying at your optimum weight is important to your success.

Dieting Leads to Disaster

There is no shortage of information being offered by the media about quick-fix foods and diet programs that will lead to weight loss. Just yesterday, while standing in a busy lineup, a glossy magazine headline caught my eye: "Fat-burning foods that can re-shape your body." I wish it were that simple.

To be frank, there are only two ways to maintain weight and reduce fat: combining healthy food choices with exercise in a slow, daily commitment to health. There is no magic formula or diet, despite the media hype and trendy, best-selling books. All one needs is a balanced diet of fruits, vegetables, whole grains, legumes, nuts, seeds, fresh juices, smoothies, and some superfoods like chlorella and spirulina. If you also add avocados, olive oil, and flax and chia seeds, you'll get your essential fatty acids and increase your high-density lipoprotein (HDL) or "good cholesterol" as a bonus.

If you combine the power of nutritious food and exercise, you'll never look back because you'll look good and feel good. That is a natural motivator.

Getting started is the hardest step.

Food, Fat Cells, and Hormones

Studies indicate that moderately obese people will slash their lifespan by up to five years while severely obese people shorten their lives by ten years or more. At best, the effects of obesity and unhealthy eating will sentence you to years of suffering from chronic illnesses and debilitating disease.

Research has shown that fat cells spew out harmful amounts of hormones and chemical reactions that break down the body. They contain an enzyme that converts adrenal steroids (androstenediol) into estrone, a form of estrogen; the higher the fat intake, the higher this conversion rate. Fat cells also aromatize testosterone into estrogen. This happens in both men and women, and it creates hormonal havoc.

The insulin resistance that comes from obesity is a major factor in degenerative diseases such as cancer, diabetes, dementia, Alzheimer's, and cardiovascular disease. If you add this hormonal imbalance to an existing, estrogen-dominant condition, which is found in many perimenopausal women, you have a known recipe for cancer. It's a perfect storm: whether it's breast cancer or another cancer, something bad will develop.

A vicious cycle occurs when too many fat cells are producing and storing too much estrogen. Estrogens are complex and powerful hormones that require a fine balance to regulate them properly. Once again, nutrition can help.

Effective estrogen eating. Some foods block estrogen; others can help the liver to purify your body of excess estrogens. Estrogen-balancing foods include the cruciferous vegetables or *Brassicas* (members of the mustard family). They include broccoli, brussel sprouts, cabbage, cauliflower, turnips, bok-choi, kohlrabi, rutabaga, and kale. These power foods detoxify excess estrogens through non-carcinogenic pathways in the liver by way of anti-cancer phytochemicals that keep your body's natural balance in top-notch form.

A large body of research has determined that estrogens are broken down into metabolites that are known to be highly carcinogenic or anticarcinogenic. The balance between the two, as measured in urine, is known as the 2/16 ratio for 2-hydroxyestrone, a weak estrogen known to be anticarcinogenic (the "good" estrogen) and 16-hydroxyestrone, which is more carcinogenic than estradiol (the "bad" estrogen). The 2-hydroxyestrone has one-tenth the estrogenic activity of 16-hydroxyestrone.

Increasing the 2-hydroxyestrone in this ratio reduces the risk of estrogen-related cancers, including breast cancer (in a 2:1 ratio) and cancers of the ovary and uterus. Recent research suggests that favorably increasing this good/bad ratio also reduces the risk of cancers of the prostate, liver, and kidney. Research has found that men in the highest third of 16-hydroxyestrone had the highest risk of prostate cancer while men in the highest third of 2-hydroxyestrone had the lowest risk.

The beauty about our metabolism is that this good/bad ratio can be modified upward just by eating moderate amounts of power foods three or four times per week. In fact, for every ten grams of cruciferous vegetables you eat each day, your good/bad ratio favorably increases by 8 percent. For those who cannot bear to eat this much cabbage, this ratio can also be raised by taking supplements of indole-3-carbinol (I3C, the phytochemical found in *Brassicas*) or preferably its downstream metabolite, 3,3'-diindolylmethane (DIM) normally formed in the stomach (each DIM molecule has 10 times the potency of an individual I3C molecule). I3C only becomes active after it's transformed into DIM by stomach acid. Since many people are low in stomach acid, it is more effective just to use DIM itself. I3C will result in a 50 percent increase in the noncarcinogenic pathway. It is very likely DIM will have a similar or even greater effect.

As well, lignans can help to balance the estrogen and progesterone ratio. Found in flax seeds, fruits (cranberries), vegetables, legumes, whole grains (rye, wheat, oat, and barley), seeds, and in the hydroxymatairesinol (HMR) derived from the Norway spruce, they help to reduce the harmful effects of excess estrogen and the formation of hormone-dependent cancers. Lignans are converted into compounds called enterolactones during metabolism by the intestinal bacteria, which research has found to offer significant cancer protection.

In women, these enterolactones reduce estrogen levels by inhibiting its binding to the sex hormone-binding globulin, which then allows estrogen to be more efficiently metabolized by the liver at a more accelerated rate. Also, enterolactone inhibits enzymes that are responsible for the conversion of estrone to estradiol, a more potent form of estrogen. Finally, studies have shown that enterolactone inhibits growth of new blood vessels into tumors and promotes cancer-cell death (apoptosis).

Eating to boost testosterone. As we'll discuss in chapter 6, exercise is the best testosterone booster, but some foods can also enhance testosterone and are often referred to as aphrodisiacs. Low levels of testosterone will inhibit sexual desire, and the mineral zinc is a proven booster of this hormone.

Adequate zinc is an important mineral for your libido. Oysters contain high levels of zinc and have long been associated with sexy foods that boost testosterone in men. Vegetarian options include baked beans and nuts.

Increasing the good/bad ratio through the consumption of cruciferous vegetables is also very beneficial to men as it reduces their risk of prostate cancer. Efficient liver metabolism, resulting in more of the weaker estrogen than the more potent one, creates less of an opportunity to bind testosterone with sex hormone-binding globulin. This increases a man's free testosterone. Lignan consumption by men is also protective, by the same mechanisms discussed above regarding women, because elevated estrogen is the culprit in the development of benign prostatic enlargement and prostate cancer.

In addition, enterolactone inhibits the aromatase enzyme that I discussed in the last chapter, which has been shown to be responsible for converting testosterone into estradiol. This has the benefit of reducing excess estrogen and boosting free testosterone. Enterolactone also inhibits another enzyme, 5-alpha reductase. This enzyme is responsible for converting testosterone to dihydrotestosterone, which has a stimulatory effect on benign and malignant prostate cells. Again, the effect is the boosting of free testosterone, which helps to reduce the risk of chronic disorders discussed in chapter 3, in addition to protecting the prostate.

Other botanicals that help to increase or preserve testosterone include Maca *(Lepidium meyenii)*, a vegetable in the broccoli family. Although it doesn't increase male sex hormones, it improves the amount still available by stimulating libido (it is a Peruvian aphrodisiac and fertility enhancer), semen quantity, and sperm quality, as well as reducing prostate enlargement in animal studies.

Muira puama *(Ptychopetalum olacoides)* is a plant used by Amazonian people to help with age-related conditions and manage stress. It enhances erectile function (in one study, 50 percent of men reported that it improved their ability to attain an erection). While its mechanism of action is still unknown, this plant contains sterols from which testosterone is made. In addition, it helps to alleviate age-related memory dysfunction through the inhibition of acetylcholinesterase, which breaks down acetylcholine, an important neurotransmitter involved in memory and cognition. It is the decline in acetylcholine levels and its receptors, particularly in the hippocampus region of the brain, that has been implicated in Alzheimer's disease.

Chrysin is a natural flavone found in many plants, especially passionflower *(Passifora incarnate)*. Although it has many benefits, including reducing anxiety, I mainly use it in patients to prevent the loss of free testosterone through inhibition of its conversion into estrogen by blocking the enzyme aromatase that causes this to happen. Because the capsule or tablet form of chrysin is not very effective, I find the best delivery system is the liposomal spray form.

Stinging nettle root *(Urtica dioica)* and ginger have shown promise in protection of the prostate through their strong anti-inflammatory activity. In particular, nettle root has been found to increase free testosterone by preventing its binding by sex hormone-binding globulin.

Low Calories, Hormones, and Aging

If you add fasting to your lifestyle, you can boost good hormones and diminish the bad ones. When I say fasting, I'm not talking about a starvation diet or a day without food. For example, if you can fast for 12 hours, four days of the week, say from 7:00 p.m. to 7:00 a.m., you will experience significant benefits to your hormones.

Consuming excess calories is very detrimental to our health. It is an independent risk factor for developing anything from cancer to vascular disease, arthritis, and even senility. Caloric restriction without malnutrition has been scientifically validated to extend the lifespan of multiple species, from microorganisms to mammals, by favoring the gene expressions leading to longevity. (For a description of how environmental factors express or suppress an inherited genetic trait, read about epigenetics in chapter 7).

Fasting actually increases production of the human growth hormone and testosterone, while decreasing the oxidative damage from cortisol and insulin. Fasting slows down the aging process by increasing the number of mitrochondria in heart and skeletal muscles, resulting in cleaner, more efficient metabolization and reduced fasting-insulin levels. Clearer skin, a taste for more nutritious foods, and an energy boost are just some of the benefits of fasting.

The positive effects of lower calories and fasting on good hormones triggers a positive response from other hormones. They are as finely interwoven as the threads in a spider's web. In addition, if you restrict your calories by 25 percent and combine an exercise program, research shows that you'll burn 15 percent more calories and also decrease the aging process by 30 percent.

If you are unable to deal with the 20 percent reduction in calories required to get the longevity benefits of caloric restriction, there are certain neutraceuticals that emulate many of the same benefits of caloric restriction. Resveratrol, pterostilbene, quercetin, and grape seed extract, along with black tea extract, appear to modulate gene expression, which protects against age-related deterioration. This is accomplished through their effects in inhibiting systemic inflammation and enhancing mitochondrial health.

Socially, Sugary Addicted

I can't talk about our food habits without talking about the "big food" major manufacturing companies and our consumption of carbonated drinks. They're loaded with high fructose corn syrup, a simple sugar that creates a calorie punch and drops our metabolism. The cliché "empty calories" is an adequate description.

These big food manufacturers have worked hard to get us addicted to their drinks and it's causing a lot of obesity in both kids and adults. Just take a look at the piles of empty beverage cans spilling out of a family's recycling box; multiply that by millions of households and you have a stark picture of our nutrition-less consumption.

Eating For a Strong Thyroid

I see thyroid imbalance every day in my practice. When you're deficient in zinc, Vitamin C, B-complex, and iodine, and your thyroid doesn't work well, you start gaining weight, become prone to insulin resistance, and suffer from a slew of other symptoms.

Many people are so deficient in iodine that their thyroids just don't work. Using iodized salt isn't enough of a remedy. This food additive has reduced the once-common incidence of goiter, or abnormally enlarged thyroid gland, which is great. However, in the 1960s the widespread use of iodine in baking bread was discontinued (because it was thought to be bad for you) and replaced with bromium.

Bromium is now in our breads, fruit and energy drinks, and vegetable oils; it actually displaces iodine in a healthy thyroid. That will create hypothyroidism by itself. This is one of the problems with convenient, processed foods: they're depleted of nutrients and, over a decade or so eating so much of it, the thyroid slows down.

Some simple, healthy foods to boost your thyroid include green vegetables. If you can't live without eating meat, use organic, wild, or free-range protein sources such as chicken, beef, salmon, and eggs. Other sources include raw nuts and seeds and fresh fruits. As well, pure, cold-pressed organic oils are hormone friendly, including extra virgin olive oil, borage, and sesame oils. But avoid all regular soy foods that contain genistein, which decreases iodine absorption. Instead, consume organic soy foods such as miso, fermented soy sauce, and fermented soy yogurts.

A whole-food, plant-based diet gives you more of those live, active nutrients to optimize and protect the thyroid. In addition, I prescribe iodine supplementation to improve thyroid functioning. A third of my patients are able to go off their thyroid medication completely; another third can reduce their dosage.

Nutraceuticals and Power Foods

I have found that this kind of nutrient supplementation can make a big difference in my patients' vitality. Their energy levels will go up on this basis alone, making them more able to increase the level of activity in their lifestyle. It's a great way to jump-start the journey back to excellent health, and it also offers sound constitutional support for the healthiest lifestyles.

Individual diets and needs vary, so consultation with a qualified professional can be invaluable both in the effectiveness and cost of the vitamins and minerals you choose. You need only walk down the aisle of your favorite pharmacy to be overwhelmed by the growing numbers of supplement choices and treatments.

Technically, vitamin and mineral supplements are still synthetic in many ways, even if they're high grade. So if you are following a high-quality diet and are not depleted in vitamins, I would recommend sticking with whole foods because it's not strictly about the vitamins. There are enzymes, proteins, and natural nutrients that, when ingested together in whole foods, enhance your body's ability to absorb all that good nutrition.

However, getting all of the necessary vitamins and minerals from whole foods can be a challenge with our typically nutrient-deficient Western diet. To determine if you are deficient in essential nutrients, a holistic health practitioner will order specific blood tests that measure various nutrient levels, such as calcium, magnesium, and Vitamin D.

Dire D-ficiency

Vitamin D is one supplement I always recommend. Even traditional medicine recognizes that Vitamin D is critical to wellness. It is estimated that if everyone had a therapeutic level of Vitamin D, it would reduce total health care costs by 25 percent. It is that important!

Studies indicate a staggering percentage of the general population is deficient in Vitamin D (the March 2010 *Journal of Clinical Endocrinology and Metabolism* reported that 59 percent of the population is deficient in Vitamin D). The risk factors for low Vitamin D levels include maturity; being female; living in northern latitudes with a long winter season; having darker skin pigmentation; a lifestyle that consists of low sunlight exposure; and dietary habits including the absence of Vitamin D fortification in common foods.

Additional factors include cultural practices where people avoid the sun and wear clothing that fully covers the skin. Individuals with cystic fibrosis or inflammatory bowel disorders such as Crohn's disease are also at high risk. There are very few foods that contain Vitamin D, and they fail to provide the daily levels required by most individuals, which adds to the challenge. The best sources of Vitamin D include the flesh of fish, such as salmon, tuna, and mackerel, and fish-oil supplements.

Deficiencies in Vitamin D are common in situations where people lack exposure to sunlight. Current estimates indicate a Vitamin D deficiency in 80 percent of residents of nursing homes, and in 40 to 100 percent of American and European elderly still living independently.

Vitamin D biochemically activates the immune system, similar to igniting the engine of a car by turning the key. In your body, Vitamin D is that key; it activates "T cells" that seek and destroy invading microorganisms as a first line of defense in your innate immune system. This occurs via genetically encoded effectors known as antimicrobial peptides (AMPs). AMPs, which are found in phagocytes and epithelial tissues, exhibit broad-spectrum antimicrobial activity against bacteria, fungi, and viruses by damaging their outer lipid membranes, rendering them vulnerable to eradication.

Current research has implicated a Vitamin D deficiency as a major factor in the pathology of at least 16 varieties of cancer as well as heart disease, stroke, hypertension, autoimmune diseases, diabetes, depression, chronic pain, osteoarthritis, osteoporosis, muscle weakness, muscle wasting, and birth defects.

The liver is responsible for converting Vitamin D2 from plant sources. Vitamin D3, or 25-hydroxyvitamin D, is mainly formed in the skin from the sun's UVB rays and from animal sources and supplements. When needed, some of the stored Vitamin D in the liver is transported to the kidneys where an enzyme converts it to its active form, 1,25-dihydroxyvitamin D, also known as calcitriol. This is the active form of Vitamin D, which has an endocrine role in regulating blood calcium when needed. When blood calcium goes up, calcitriol goes down and when blood calcium goes down, calcitriol goes up.

Although important for calcium regulation due to calcium's role in optimizing muscle and nerve functioning, calcitriol shines in its function as a molecular switch that turns on 2000 target genes (10 percent of the human genome). This unique ability to switch cell functions on and off prevents uncontrolled growth of potentially cancerous cells while stimulating cells to differentiate (mature) so that they can carry out their prime functions. Through this molecular control, calcitriol has a dual effect on the immune system. That is, it can boost deficient immune function and quiet an overactive immune system. It is protective against cancers and autoimmune diseases.

Vitamin D also reduces inflammation and oxidative damage that have been implicated in conditions such as osteoarthritis, chronic obstructive pulmonary disease, cardiovascular disease, and metabolic syndrome. This is why it is so important to get yearly 25-hydroxyvitamin D blood levels checked as these mechanisms depend on having sufficient amounts of this storage hormone to access when needed.

There are many organs in the body that have Vitamin D receptors, including the brain, prostate, breasts, and colon, as well as cells involved in immunity and genetic regulation. Receptors also exist in skeletal muscles. One of the most common symptoms of Vitamin D deficiency is muscle weakness and soreness. Many people diagnosed with fibromyalgia and chronic-fatigue syndrome suffer from aches and pains associated with this deficiency. In addition, research into muscle weakness and an increased likelihood of falling include five randomized studies representing 1237 participants. Supplementing with 800 international units (IU) per day of Vitamin D significantly reduced the incidence of falling by 22 percent.

Cognitive function is improved with Vitamin D supplementation. Recent European studies show that men with higher Vitamin D levels performed better in tests of attention and the speed of their information processing. Vitamin D supplementation is also shown to reduce the incidence of multiple sclerosis by 42 percent; the incidence of Type I diabetes by 80 percent; and Type II diabetes by 33 percent.

Research also indicates lower risks of lymphoma as well as colon, pancreatic, ovarian, and breast cancers with higher levels of Vitamin D. Congestive heart failure, elevated c-reactive protein in the blood (an indication of inflammation), schizophrenia, depression, and respiratory wheezing have all been linked to Vitamin D deficiency.

If you have a history of osteoporosis, a bone scan will show you the areas affected; you will likely need some calcium and magnesium, in addition to Vitamin D. I also strongly advise bioidentical hormone therapy, such as progesterone, which enhances calcium absorption and not only prevents bone loss but actually builds bone.

The American Journal of the Medical Sciences reported that Vitamin D deficiency is associated with high blood pressure, heart failure, and ischemic heart disease. Patients with heart failure, especially African Americans, are prone to an imbalance of several nutrients. Studies suggest that managing this condition should include supplementing with calcium, magnesium, zinc, selenium, Vitamins B12 and B1, as well as Vitamin D.

Such research into the role of nutrition in the causation, prevention, and treatment of cardiovascular disease will undoubtedly open up new treatment frontiers by identifying simple remedies that could advance the study of the practice of medicine.

How much to take? The U.S.-based, independent Institute of Medicine (the health-advisor arm of the National Academy of Sciences) recommends supplementing with 200 IU of Vitamin D per day; patients between the ages of 51 and 70 should take 400 IU per day, and those over the age of 70 should take 600 IU per day. Many wellness physicians (myself included) know these dosages are insufficient to meet the body's needs for proper Vitamin D activity.

A 25-hydroxyvitamin D blood test is required to diagnose Vitamin D deficiency and (at least annually) to monitor the change in blood levels with ongoing, therapeutic supplementation on a regular basis. I will prescribe Vitamin D3 at 2000 to 5000 IU per day, depending on the level of deficiency indicated. I find that 90 percent of individuals will require 5000 IU of Vitamin D with approximately 5 percent requiring 10,000 IU and the other 5 percent needing about 2000 IU to reach my target: a therapeutic 25-hydroxy blood level between 50 and 80 ng/ml.

Higher dosages may be required if you weigh more than 180 pounds. Heavier people require more Vitamin D. And if you are over the age of 55, you need a higher dose because less Vitamin D is converted in the skin from sunlight as we age. Children will require 1000 IU of Vitamin D for every 25 lb of body weight.

Research published over the last decade suggests that Vitamin D toxicity is unlikely at daily intake levels of 10,000 IU or less. I always prefer Vitamin D3 (cholecalciferol) over Vitamin D2 (ergocalciferol) supplementation. Vitamin D2 is about 20 to 40 percent as effective as Vitamin D3 in maintaining serum concentrations of 25-dihydroxyvitamin D because it is more rapidly broken down in the body.

Care must be used in taking supplements with excess levels of preformed Vitamin A because it competes with Vitamin D at the receptor site, thereby blocking the beneficial effects of Vitamin D. Preformed Vitamin A is "active retinol" as opposed to "beta-carotene," which converts to retinol in the body on demand (beta-carotene is not a problem). Most multivitamin formulations and modern cod liver oil have a ratio of ten times more Vitamin A than Vitamin D, thereby thwarting Vitamin D's protective effects and leading to increased mortality. You should avoid supplements with excess preformed Vitamin A (take only 500 to 1000 IU per day) and ensure adequate amounts of Vitamin D.

Other Power Nutrients

Since there are volumes of books on the subject of vitamins, I will not reinvent the wheel. But here are a few examples from recent research that you may not have come across.

It turns out that mom was right when she insisted that we eat our fruits and vegetables. The U.S. Department of Health has recommended for years to eat at least five portions of fruits and vegetables in our daily diet but this recommendation is steadily increasing to up to 13 servings, depending on one's caloric intake. However, 33 percent of American adults eat only two servings of fruits and vegetables per day, with half the population eating no fruit at all.

Why eat fruits and vegetables? There is compelling evidence that fruits and vegetables protect us from chronic diseases through their antioxidant ability. They lower the risk of heart disease and stroke (people eating more than five servings daily lower their risk by 20 percent compared to people eating less than three servings per day). They help to control blood pressure and protect against certain cancers (carotenoids may protect against lung, mouth, prostate, and throat cancer). In addition, because they contain indigestible fiber, they will calm an irritable bowel by triggering bowel movements, preventing constipation, diverticulosis, and diverticulitis. A diet rich in fruits and vegetables (particularly lutein and zeaxanthin found in dark green leafy vegetables) reduces the chances of developing cataracts or macular degeneration in our eyes, which are exquisitely sensitive to the damaging effects of free radicals generated by sunlight, cigarette smoke, air pollution, infection, and metabolism.

The problem with ingesting so many fruits and vegetables is pesticide contamination from these foods. You can make informed choices to lower your dietary pesticide load by following the guidelines from the most recent 2010 Environmental Working Group (EWF) shoppers' guide to pesticides (see Table 4.1). This list informs you of the 12 most contaminated fruits and vegetables (therefore, only buy organic) and the 15 that are lowest in pesticides. Research indicates that people who eat five fruits and vegetables a day from the "dirty dozen" side will consume an average of ten pesticides a day. Fewer than two pesticides daily will be consumed with the "clean fifteen" side of the list.

Table 4.1:   Shoppers' Guide to Pesticides from the Environmental Working Group

Dirty Dozen (the worst, so buy organic)	Clean 15 (lowest in pesticides)
1. Celery (worst)	1. Onions (best)
2. Peaches	2. Avocado
3. Strawberries	3. Sweet corn
4. Apples	4. Pineapple
5. Blueberries	5. Mangoes
6. Nectarines	6. Sweet peas
7. Bell peppers	7. Asparagus

8.	Spinach	8.	Kiwi
9.	Kale	9.	Cabbage
10.	Cherries	10.	Eggplant
11.	Potatoes	11.	Cantaloupe
12.	Grapes (imported)	12.	Watermelon
		13.	Grapefruit
		14.	Sweet potato
		15.	Honeydew melon

Essential fatty acids (EFAs) are essential to human health but cannot be made by the body, so they must be provided from our food. They are required to help build the membranes in all cells, strengthen immune cells, help lubricate joints, provide energy, prevent skin from drying out, and a host of other functions. The two EFA families are omega-3 and omega-6.

Omega-3 EFAs include eicosapentaenoic acid (EPA) and docosahexaenoic acid (DHA) and are found in fish oils, nuts, and olive oil. Flax seed, hemp, walnut, and soybean oils contain an omega-3 called alpha-linolenic acid (ALA), which can be converted into EPA, and then into DHA. The omega-6 fatty acids, linoleic acid (LA) and gamma-linolenic acid (GLA), are found in the seeds of borage, evening primrose, sunflower, and black currant plants.

As many as 96,000 people die each year in the United States due to lack of omega-3s in their diets, according to research led by the Harvard School of Public Health. On the other hand, getting sufficient omega-3s offers multiple benefits, including a longer life, overall improved health, a leaner physique, a clearer head, and younger-looking skin. The beneficial effects of omega-3 fatty acids are well known for their anti-inflammatory effect throughout the whole body. Dr. Joseph Maroon, author of *Fish Oil: The Natural Anti-inflammatory*, believes that fish oils modulate genetic expression by activating DNA to "reduce inflammation, reduce cancer formation, protect from clot formation, and improve nerve cell communications." They improve brain function, reduce Alzheimer's disease, reduce the risk of heart attacks by 28 percent and sudden cardiac death by 25 percent, reduce the risk of ischemic strokes, improve the outcome of autoimmune diseases, and improve vision. For example, the *Archives of Ophthalmology* reveal that patients who consumed one serving of fish per week had a 31 percent lower risk of developing early macular degeneration. Recent evidence also links omega-3 EFAs with decreasing the risk of developing type 1 diabetes. See Table 4.2 for specific benefits.

Table 4.2:	Therapeutic Value of Omega-3s
Reduced risk for heart disease	
Relief from inflammatory diseases	
Higher levels of HDL (good cholesterol)	
Lower levels of LDL (bad cholesterol)	
Lower levels of triglycerides (elevated levels increase health risks)	
Less likelihood of high blood pressure	
Reduced risk of artery-clogging plaque or blood clots	
After a heart attack, less risk of sudden death from another heart attack of stroke	
Improved blood sugar control among people who are overweight	
Less joint pain and stiffness among people with arthritis	
Improved bone health	
Improved mood	
Less hostility and improved overall function among children with attention deficit or hyperactivity disorders	
Improved healing of skin conditions such as psoriasis	
Reduced sensitivity to the sun	
Reduction of asthma symptoms among children	
Lower risk of macular degeneration	
Relief from PMS and menopausal symptoms	
Reduced risk for colon cancer and possibly breast and prostate cancers	
Healthy development of the neurological system in the womb and among infants and children	

Studies have shown that most of the neurological benefits of omega-3 oils are derived from the DHA component rather than the EPA component. DHA makes up 50 percent of the retina's structure, which is why it prevents macular degeneration. It makes up 30 percent of the brain, and plays a major role in brain development of the fetus and during the first two years of life. Dr David Perlmutter, in his book *How to Raise a Smarter Child by Kindergarten,* believes that a child's IQ can be raised by as much as 30 points, in part by supplementing with DHA in the critical first three years. In addition, DHA impacts behavior in a positive way; it supports healthy levels of neurotransmitters (promoting focused attention and calming anxiety), improves chronic depression, and reduces aggressive behavior. It will also decrease plasma norepinephrine levels, thus reducing the stress response. For the above reasons, omega-3 oils must be considered a mainstay of any diet. In a supplemental regimen, care must be taken to ensure that your omega-3 EFAs come from a high-quality fish oil product; less expensive "over-the-counter" products contain significant amounts of PCBs and mercury.

The leaves from olive trees have been used medicinally since ancient times. Supplements containing olive tree extracts can help to lower blood pressure and cholesterol. Their excellent antiviral properties help to fight numerous forms of influenza.

Cabbage is a powerful nutrient compound. Research indicates that cabbage can heal duodenal ulcers in a third of the usual time by strengthening patients' stomach lining to make it more resistant to acid attacks. Eating cabbage is sometimes called the "anti-ulcer U factor." The active ingredient, glutamine, is also available in capsules; it has proven to be more effective than antacids.

Many studies are proving the benefits of probiotic bacteria. These microorganisms, found throughout the intestinal tract, are part of its natural ecology. They help to digest food and kill harmful microorganisms; research indicates that levels of these "friendly" bacteria decline as we age. In addition, the role of these friendly intestinal bacteria flora is to occupy the intestinal tract, thus preventing the unfriendly bacteria and other organisms from becoming predominant. If the latter occurs, inflammation of the bowels and other disorders arise. Taking antibiotics for infections will indiscriminately kill good and bad bacteria alike, leaving the intestinal tract vulnerable to the overgrowth of unfriendly bacteria. A quality probiotic supplement will reintroduce the friendly bacteria into our digestive systems, creating a barrier on the intestinal wall that stops the unfriendly bacteria from invading cells.

Taking supplemental probiotic bacteria can dramatically reduce the rate of Candida and other yeast infections. Recent studies also reveal that eating seven ounces of yogurt containing live lactobacilli bacteria can significantly reduce the number of respiratory and nasal infections.

Green tea is now well known for its antioxidant properties, but you won't absorb about 80 percent of what you drink. The active ingredient that lowers your risk for chronic diseases (and offers glucose control) quickly loses its power in your intestines. Boost absorption by adding freshly squeezed lemon, orange, lime, or grapefruit juice to your tea. The Vitamin C aids absorption by increasing the cilia in the small intestine.

Human and animal studies have reported that eating diets rich in grapes, berries, and walnuts can help to preserve brain function and memory in older individuals. The chemicals in these foods contain a wide range of anti-cancer, anti-inflammatory, and antioxidant properties.

Your Power Tool

I can't stress enough that your fork is your greatest power tool for remaining healthy and strong throughout the years of your life. Eating better is the greatest way to improve your overall well-being and recapture your youthful vigor. It sounds so simple, but I know that it's not easy. I hear you! I have to deal with it, too: the pull Ronald McDonald exerts on my children, with his prizes and playground, can be irresistible.

In today's rushed world, most people are experiencing the same challenges. How do you find the time to exercise, eat or prepare nutritious food, and allow for down time? But the influence of food and lifestyle is so important to our health that 80 percent of chronic illness may be caused by the combination of a poor diet and a stressful, sedentary lifestyle.

As I always say to my patients, there's no such thing as a "fountain of youth" pill; there's just a "fountain of youth" lifestyle. That means you have to make healthier food choices and implement permanent changes into your diet. You must also manage your stress, and fit exercise into your schedule. If you sincerely want to age with grace and health, there's your magic formula.

The solution is simple. Well, maybe not so simple. But it is essential for aging to perfection. The next two chapters will discuss the effects of stress and exercise on your body, mind, and spirit as you reach the height of your mature power and wisdom.

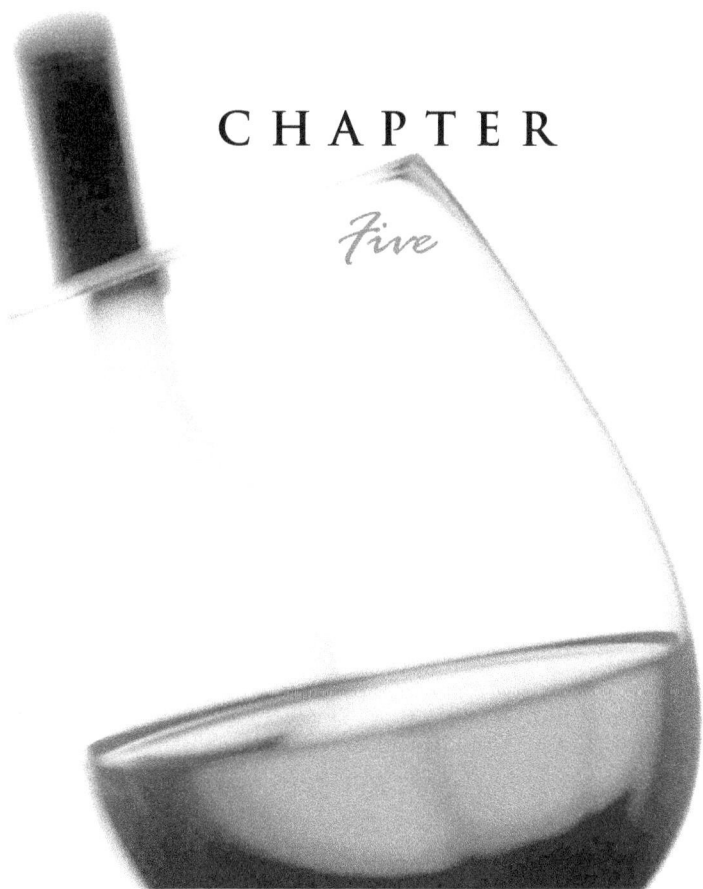

CHAPTER

Five

CHAPTER FIVE

Stress Speeds Aging

"In the central place of every heart there is a
recording chamber. So long as it receives a message of beauty,
hope, cheer, and courage - so long are you young. When the wires
are all down and our heart is covered with the snow of
pessimism and the ice of cynicism, then,
and only then, are you grown old."

D o u g l a s   M a c A r t h u r

Ongoing, unrelieved stress literally eats your brain! Studies prove this. It doesn't matter whether it's physiological, biological, mental, emotional, nutritional, or environmental stress; it all has the same result. Unrelenting stress is as equal in its capacity to seriously harm you as the most toxic environmental pollutant. It overloads the brain with powerful hormones that are intended only for short-term duty in emergency situations. Their cumulative effect damages and kills brain cells and wreaks havoc with your physical, mental, and emotional balance.

When you encounter a threat, your body reacts by increasing your adrenaline flow, tensing muscles, and ramping up your heart and respiration rates. Cortisol, which is secreted by the adrenal glands, converts amino acids into glucose energy, enhances your memory functions, lowers your sensitivity to pain, and supports your immune system. All of these functions constitute the biological wiring meant to assist you in dealing with a "fight or flight" situation. When the threat ends, these functions are ramped back down.

The problem is that today's stress is unrelenting. Modern man is under stress constantly, from the rushed breakfast spent coordinating family schedules to the pressures of the work day and well into the evening as we strive to complete all the tasks scheduled into our day. Stress never stops, and it's killing us.

The book *Why Zebras Don't Get Ulcers* details the difference between how we experience stress and what happens in the natural world. Out on the Serengeti plains, stress occurs when a lion chases you. It's a one-time response. The flight-or-fight reaction happens for a brief period of time and then it goes away. Afterward, the animals graze as if nothing happened. But as humans, we don't regulate ourselves regarding stress. We don't dial down.

Unrelenting stress causes cortisol to continue pouring into your bloodstream and the consequences are highly destructive. They include impaired cognitive performance in terms of concentration, memory, and problem solving; suppressed thyroid function, causing blood-sugar imbalances that lead to insulin resistance; decreases in bone density and muscle tissue; elevated blood pressure; and increased abdominal fat, which leads to assorted health risks such as heart attacks and strokes.

It can also lower your immunity, slow wound healing, and increase inflammatory responses in the body that lead to age-related, degenerative diseases. Behaviorally, emotions such as anxiety, irritability, sadness, and depression, or even extreme happiness and exhilaration, are paired with reduced physical control, insomnia, and irrational actions.

Stress activates the sympathetic nervous system, which is responsible for up- and down-regulation of many homeostatic mechanisms. The hippocampus, located in the brain, activates this process. Studies show a connection between long-lasting stress and erosion of its functioning.

Because the hippocampus is thought to play a central role in memory, there has been considerable interest in the connection between hippocampal atrophy and age-related diseases. It is one of the earliest signs of Alzheimer's disease; it is associated with memory loss and mood disorders; and it is present in patients with post-traumatic stress disorder, schizophrenia, and severe depression.

If you remove the source of your stress, the hippocampus will grow back. But this takes a concerted effort to live a much less-stressful lifestyle. You can learn to relax your body with various techniques, make changes to your diet and exercise level, and cultivate healthy, emotional and mental attitudes. All of these can help to buffer the effect of stress on your immune functioning and overall health.

Any stressor immediately leads to a six-hour shutdown of the immune system. If it is unresolved, you will most certainly get sick. Add two events together, such as eating a donut (diet stress) in your car on the way to work and then yelling at a lousy driver (emotional stress), and you will earn a 12-hour shutdown of your immune system. Bereavement leads to discombobulating the whole body for as much as six months.

Just reading a horror story or watching the evening news can compromise your health, depending on how you experience it. The brain has the ability to selectively activate the fight-or-flight responses and people are biologically "wired" to react differently to stress.

One person may secrete higher levels of cortisol than another in the same situation. Our individual ability to handle stress has much to do with our genetics, personality type, and environmental influences. Early childhood trauma can significantly increase a person's stress response. Scientists have recognized that stress in childhood or early life can create a hyper-vigilancy and hyper-response to stressors later in life.

Stress will diminish all of your critical sex hormones. With chronic stress, eventually the adrenals are exhausted and production of these important hormones is drastically reduced. Progesterone declines when the body favors cortisol to reduce the stress; over time, the result is a serious deficit in progesterone. Stress is also one of the most frequently overlooked causes of estrogen dominance in women; men will experience a decrease in testosterone.

As you age, you must be more careful about how you handle stress because the burden on your body is greater. Age-related declines in hormone levels, increased inflammation in the body, and the accumulation of toxins makes it that much more difficult to recover from long-term stress. Like the straw that breaks the camel's back, it can add up until you break down.

To remain youthfully active with a strong, healthy constitution, you want to ensure that your mental faculties, muscles, moods, and every part of yourself are in prime condition.

Where the body goes, the mind follows: if you deliberately work to reduce your physical stress response, your mind will de-stress. Exercise, yoga, deep-breathing exercises, and sex are all helpful in relieving stress. Bodywork therapies, such as massage and Reiki energy work, are also proven to be effective.

Where the mind goes, the body follows: certain mental practices will reduce the stress in your body.

Where the mind goes, the body follows: certain mental practices will reduce the stress in your body. If you entertain thoughts and images of health and well-being, you can expect your parasympathetic nervous system, which is in control of the relaxation response, to give the all-clear signal and your glands and organs will function as necessary when life is good.

Meditation and guided imagery, and the cultivation of a positive, optimistic mental attitude, foster emotional resilience. You also have the ability to affect the amount of stress you experience through your perception of stress. A lively, buoyant optimism will help you to overcome challenges without being deeply affected by them.

Music that heals the body and soul is another known de-stressor, and it has a lot of psychological benefits. It reduces pain and anxiety, and improves your ability to sleep. Studies show that Alzheimer's patients connect through music when they cannot connect verbally with people.

Mikala's Miracle

The following story is a good illustration of the physical, mental, and emotional issues that come with unrelieved stress. As a busy mother of two teenage boys, and a full-time teacher, Mikala Vonn was used to an energetic, active lifestyle until multiple stressors added up to sap her vitality. "Life was rich, full, and very rewarding," she says of the days before both her parents died. After that, the stressors just kept on coming.

Increasing family demands included some sibling issues; meanwhile, she completed a Master's degree at the age of 52. However, a political upheaval at her school added another layer of stress. All of these stressors, combined together, eroded her capacity to handle her responsibilities.

"I began to experience more and more physical issues," she recalls. These included menstrual periods that lasted six weeks, and plummeting energy levels; she experienced anxiety attacks, an inability to sleep at night, and myriad other physical ailments.

When medical tests revealed an enlarged ovary and uterine polyp, she was referred to a specialist for "a regimen of biopsies, the standard drug interventions, and a final result of more 'abnormal cells' present. It was the suspected hint of 'cancer' that led to a hysterectomy in 2007."

Left with one ovary, she was told that hormone replacement therapy (HRT) would not be required. "Artificial HRT supplements were available in every size and color if I needed them. I was skeptical about the artificial supplements and all their potential health risks. I had just been given a new lease on life, so why would I risk any further exposure to ingredients that could possibly lead to more cancer risks!"

But her hormones were now in chaos. Insomnia became the norm. "I noticed changes in my ability to concentrate, feeling overwhelmed by everyday tasks, difficulty remembering details, weight gain, fatigue, and foggy thinking. I got more and more upset at what I was feeling, unable to control any of it."

"I took over-the-counter sleep aids and herbal teas, but nothing helped me sleep," she says. "Excessive amounts of stress and anxiety increased. I felt more and more helpless and depressed. I knew something was wrong!"

After hearing about bioidentical hormones on the Oprah Winfrey show, she added this information to her growing dossier on alternative treatments. "I didn't relate the intensity of my symptoms to hormonal intervention until a dear friend of mine, who had also experienced similar physical issues, encouraged me to go have my hormone levels checked."

Mikala knew the conventional methods of hormone testing wouldn't be good enough, nor was she willing to take synthetic drugs. "I was convinced that the natural alternatives were the best option for me," she says.

"Dr. Garcia was encouraging, knowledgeable, and very 'in tune' with the issues surrounding my physical symptoms. He did a complete battery of tests on me, including saliva, to check my hormone levels. I was shocked at the outcome." Mikala was suffering from adrenal fatigue and a progesterone deficiency.

"My cortisol levels were extremely high in the morning, exposing my prolonged insomnia issues. The risk of long-term health problems as a result of these symptoms, including diabetes and heart disease, scared me to death! I wanted to be vital, happy, and healthy again," she says.

A regimen of nutraceuticals and bioidentical hormones began to deliver after just one month. "I began to feel less anxious and depressed, more energetic, started sleeping for longer periods of time, and felt a sense of hope that, finally, there would be relief from my physical ailments. At the end of three months, I was feeling a remarkable difference in myself. I was actually dreaming again, had less foggy thinking, was remembering more, and feeling more optimistic for the first time in a long time."

Six months later, she reported feel "balanced" and "normal" again, with good memory skills. "Insomnia has almost disappeared, and I feel like my old self. I no longer feel overwhelmed and I have more energy to engage in my life again. How my life has changed for the better!"

Mikala says that her treatment of nutraceutical supplements and bioidentical hormones returned "my health, life, and sense of well-being." Her friends and family noticed quite a difference. "Everyone has noticed that the 'old, vital me' has returned. I am thrilled, too! I now have a renewed sense of optimism and hope for the future."

Getting Enough Sleep

To regain hormonal balance, you must first normalize the adrenal gland. In fact, bioidentical replacement of deficient hormones alone, without addressing the overall health of the adrenal gland, is ineffective over the long term. The normalization process begins with stress reduction. This includes relaxation and rest, and getting enough sleep.

Adrenal fatigue can arise just from not sleeping well. I would say, conservatively, that 90 percent of the women, and 70 percent of the men, I see have sleep problems. Without good-quality sleep, you will never restore your adrenals.

Certain nutraceuticals offer natural sleep aids, including tryptophan, a precursor to serotonin; magnesium (citrate or glycinate), which helps you to relax; and melatonin, which is produced by the pineal gland. You may be able to improve your quality of sleep by simply avoiding substances that affect your sleep. This includes not drinking coffee after 6:00 p.m. and having nothing to drink just before you go to sleep.

Another strategy is avoiding all light in your room, including your clock's dial. Reducing electromagnetic frequencies in the bedroom has helped many people. This includes moving electrical clocks, radios, and television sets away from your bed because they can disrupt your sleep.

Good sleep hygiene is about restoring the body's natural circadian rhythms. This is done by going to bed at the same time each night and getting up every day at the same time.

Physical Resilience

Good nutrition supports your body's functioning as well as your entire body-mind-spirit connection in dealing with life's stressors. A plant-based, organic diet helps to nourish every cell with the essential ingredients for optimal functioning.

The physical stressors in our environment are considerable, and often unavoidable. Breathing the air is stressful because it contains many carcinogenic compounds; if you smoke cigarettes, you only add to this burden. We drink polluted water. We consume beverages loaded with sugar and artificial chemicals, and we over-consume caffeine and alcohol. Dietary stress comes from eating processed foods barren of nutrients. Our food supply is loaded with toxins such as mercury, which is present in almost all fish. This stresses the body, weakening it and opening the way for diseases.

Another way to help your body handle stress with strength and wholeness is to restore hormonal balance. Think of bioidentical hormones as a large branch of your tree of health. They naturally support every part of your functioning, with an enhanced sense of well-being that goes down to the cellular level. In addition to physical vitality, this can benefit you mentally and spiritually because of how balanced your life feels.

Bioidentical testosterone therapy improves depression, builds muscle mass, and enhances endurance. A testosterone deficiency leads to what I call the "grumpy older men syndrome": it physically and mentally ruins a man's overall quality of life. Cases of depression are also connected to low levels of T3 thyroid hormone, and women with low estrogen levels can also exhibit signs of depression. (This is often illustrated by the "blues" that accompany estrogen dips as part of a woman's menstrual cycle. It foreshadows the kind of trouble a woman will experience during menopause).

I have found that, with bioidentical hormone supplementation, my patients start feeling better and looking better, and this in itself is a stress reliever. Their whole outlook and attitude changes; they start going out more, and not isolating themselves. They feel physically stronger and healthier. Where the body goes, the mind follows: it's all connected.

We are genetically disposed to certain chronic diseases through inherited physiological traits. Whether or not we actually experience that disease is determined in part by our parents. However, our health is also affected by the food we eat, the exercise we do, the unaddressed stressors we tolerate, the toxins we permit into our body, and the quality of our hormonal balance. We are not resigned to our own genetic predisposition; we can actually alter it. These choices are as individually unique as our fingerprints.

How people react to stress is a factor of how they are raised. It's very similar to the hygiene hypothesis: if you are not exposed to viruses or bacteria before the age of two, you may have lifelong problems with your immune system. As parents, we want to prevent our children from having illnesses or viruses when young, but exposure is actually important for developing the immune system so that it can handle diseases in the future. In the same way, the ability to handle stress depends on how we were exposed to it at a younger age.

Too much stress in childhood can be detrimental, but too little stress can also inhibit the effectiveness of our mature response. Our ability to deal as adults is based on how we dealt with stress in childhood. The extent to which hormones such as adrenalin and cortisol are elevated during a stressful event is connected to the way we meet the challenges we face.

The mind-body connection is the real deal. During meditation, Tibetan monks are able to stimulate their own vagus nerve and relax deeply, reducing their heart rate and breathing. You can do it, too. The vagus nerve is part of the parasympathetic nervous system. It helps to regulate your heartbeat, controls muscle movement, helps to keep you breathing, and transmits a variety of chemicals throughout your body. It is also responsible for keeping your digestive tract in working order, contracting the muscles of the stomach and intestines to help process food, and sending back information about what is being digested and what the body is getting out of it.

If you stimulate this nerve, it releases the feel-good neurotransmitter acetylcholine. It is this chemical that balances the stressful effects of adrenalin and cortisol from the sympathetic nervous system by activating the relaxation response. It douses the molecular wildfire created by adrenalin and cortisol through its calming, anti-inflammatory effect when the vagus nerve is stimulated. The good news is that you can activate this relaxation response whenever you want because you are in control.

You can stimulate the vagus nerve using Tibetan monk-like meditation techniques but it is much simpler to do deep belly breathing several times a day. One of my favorite techniques, which is also extremely easy to learn, is the emotional freedom technique (emofree.com).

There are many ways to activate this relaxation response and not one technique is better than another. But you must find the one that works for you. It may be prayer, exercise, music, dancing, laughter, human connection, bubble baths, massage, yoga, or saunas. The net effect will be the same: it will stop inflammation by reducing the stress hormones. Then your brain and body can begin to heal and repair.

Natural Harmony

Have you ever wondered why people feel better about themselves and their fellow travelers after a long walk in the woods? It's the connection to nature that is the reason we want to get out of the rat race. As comedienne Lily Tomlin once observed, the trouble with the rat race is that the winners are still rats.

We know that we live in an artificial world of concrete and metal and it tends to make us forget about the emotional intimacy that comes from being naturally connected. This is exactly what has been seen in a study from Rochester, New York, where exposure to nature influenced people to be more thoughtful of others and less concerned about self. Other studies have shown the health benefits of nature, ranging from rapid healing to powerful stress reduction to increased mental performance and physical vitality.

The study showed that nature brings out more sociable feelings, with more value placed on community and close relationships. People are more caring when they are surrounded by nature. People immersed in natural environments report a higher value in intrinsic aspirations, deep and durable relationships, and a commitment to working toward the betterment of society.

There was also an attendant lowering of the perceived value of expensive, material aspirations such as financial success or being admired by many people. It showed that a connection to nature can boost your inclination to cooperate rather than compete and doing good instead of merely looking good.

Refocusing your values is extremely stress-reducing. To rebalance your life, consider a long nature walk or just go outdoors for a while. You can recreate these good effects indoors with symbolic reminders of the outside life such as houseplants, paintings, photographs, gardens visible from your window, and even natural screensavers on your computer.

You don't have to take a vacation to Alaska to enjoy nature; you can be a bird watcher, a hiker, a gardener, or a landscape artist. The health effects of being out in nature can also apply to hunters, trappers, and fishermen. You can also paint natural scenes or take photographs of nature.

Cushion Against Stress

Another extremely powerful anti-stress practice is building a margin of time into your daily life. In our fast-paced world, we continually race from obligation to deadline to appointment to activity, often with split-second timing and no room for error. It can be a performance worthy of an Olympic medal. If you do it over and over again, day after day, this can lead to your destruction instead of success.

Just making it to that movie with five minutes to spare adds to your stress load. Building in a cushion of time between all of your commitments gives you a margin of room that allows you to approach life in a more relaxed fashion. It helps you to deal with stress. Schedule time to complete your tasks and spend time with your loved ones in such a way that you feel less rushed. It is a way of supporting yourself throughout your day.

If you're typically a hard-charging person, always packing your schedule with too much activity and fighting upstream all the day long, then slow down and give yourself time to enjoy life. Stand outside your car for a moment and enjoy the look of the sun and sky, or gaze at the stars. Aim for quality time to enjoy everything you do. It's the little, least expensive things in life that are the most precious.

Support yourself in this sort of way by allowing ample time to get from place to place or just stop for a while and be. This sort of practice helps you to build self-worth in everything you do, and its value is beyond your ability to calculate.

Emotional Support

Social support is an important factor in helping people to live longer. As The Blue Zones showed, the longest-lived people actively value their connection to others. Without this, people will die sooner. It gives you a sense of purpose and control over your world; you feel connected to others, and valued enough to be included. It creates a sense of optimism about your world and builds your self-esteem. Studies show that social interaction even helps wounds to heal faster.

Instead of stepping on everyone to get ahead, which is an incredibly stressful practice, cultivate compassion for others and a softer heart. This can lead to less stress in your life; what you give out truly does come back to you, and it is better to give than receive. The small things you do will ultimately make you feel better about yourself and leave you wanting to do even more.

According to the study of genomics, you are the sum total of all your experiences, both good and bad. When it comes to stress, unresolved trauma from the past will echo forward into your present and add to your stress load. If something bad happened, it can carry through your life to affect your future. Letting go of the past is a powerful stress buster.

To start with, you must learn to forgive. Writings throughout the ages and many alternative healing therapies bring to light that unresolved emotions can manifest as disease on the cellular level in the physical body. Not forgiving makes you sick. The whole biblical concept about forgiveness is true. You have to forgive if you want to live, especially yourself. Shake off that guilt complex and let go of what has happened. Letting go of negative thoughts is the first step in the healing journey.

The toughest person to forgive is yourself. People who think that they're not worthy tend to sabotage their own success through this belief. You have to get over it, whatever it is you think that you've done or not done. Let go of the past to have a healthy present and future.

Another healthy attitude is giving up competing with your inner self. We all have an internal value system, and sometimes it is very dysfunctional. If you are working under a tremendous performance burden, where you feel internal pressure to be a certain way and produce to certain standards, it can cause a great deal of stress in your life. Add to this a subconscious belief that you will ultimately fail in your endeavors and you have a double-stress recipe.

Attitude Adjustment

I believe that cancer develops because of the negative things we harbor. It creates the same physiological stress. Eventually it makes you sick. If you're the kind of person who sees the glass as half empty, then your negative feelings are contributing to a chronic inflammatory condition in your body. This inflammatory cascade will quickly age you.

You have to change your attitude. When it comes to negative learned behaviors, unlearn them! If your thinking has been channeled down the same negative path, take the next fork and open up your optimism and your lifestyle for greater vitality. A one-way street to illness can become a two-way street to health.

Living a less stressful, healthier life, where you feel a surfeit of energy and boundless enthusiasm for your days, depends on the choices you make. The attitude you choose to bring to every situation is critical to your body-mind-spirit connection. No matter what the challenge, unresolved family issues, problems with a boss at work, chronic health issues, you can overcome it with the right attitude.

During World War II, Viktor Frankl, a Jewish psychiatrist, was thrown into prison by the Nazis. His father, mother, brother, and wife died in the camps or were sent to the ovens. He lived from day to day, every hour expecting to be killed by his Nazi tormentors. Then one day, naked and alone in his small cell, he became aware of the one freedom they could not take away: his right to decide within himself how to respond to what they did.

He survived four Nazi camps, including Auschwitz, and went on to become Europe's leading psychiatrist with 32 books published and translated into 26 languages. He wrote, "Everything can be taken from a man, but one thing; the last of the human freedoms, to choose one's attitudes, in any given set of circumstances, to choose one's own way." If anyone should have developed an angry, unforgiving, depressed attitude, it was this man. But he chose optimism in the face of tragedy and is an example of the human potential within everyone, including you.

How you respond to the curveballs that life throws at you, no matter how bad they are, is determined within yourself. Choose a healthy attitude and you will find healing. No one said this is easy, but choosing the Frankl path helps you to make that first step toward greater health and will make an impact on your happiness and, by extension, your longevity.

The right attitude makes it easier to jump the hurdles in life, and an important one is taking responsibility for yourself and your actions. If you constantly think of yourself as a victim, to whom life is being unfair, this position of helplessness will immobilize you and inhibit your ability to act effectively. Okay, so you didn't get the job or promotion, or your spouse asks for a divorce; take responsibility for yourself and use this to change the way you look at life.

Stop operating from self-pity and an obsession about what is wrong. Look at what is going right in your life. If you really think that you have a difficult life, walk with me through the children's cancer ward of your local hospital. You'll see so much innocent suffering that you won't ever pity your own life again. Come from a position of gratitude and it will change your attitude.

There is a lot of interest in mental imagery's ability to help people live a successful, high-quality life. It is a popular tool, widely used in many professions such as the financial industry and team sports. The image you hold in your subconscious mind can determine your level of performance. It helps to build a bridge between your subconscious and conscious mind so that they are both on the same wavelength and neither is sabotaging your wishes.

The imagery is important; you start by creating a visual template of what you want in life, and then use it to achieve the outcome you desire. By concentrating on the image, you are communicating to your subconscious mind what you want. Proponents of this technique say it is astonishingly effective.

After all, if you were traveling in France but did not know the language, you could still communicate by showing someone a picture of what you want. The same is true of talking with your subconscious mind. By concentrating on that image, your subconscious mind will then know the language that you're talking, and can strive for what you want.

No matter what your goal, a house, a car, or greater health, positive mental imagery can help you to achieve it. You can also use this technique to build healthier relationships.

A Merry Heart

Cultivate optimism about life; this in itself will protect you against stress-related health problems. Give away your negative emotions and stay firmly rooted within a positive attitude about your life. This is what I call a merry heart, and it is a powerful tool for longevity.

Laughter promotes a sense of well-being and stimulates your internal organs. People who can't laugh, who hate their job, their spouse, and their status in life, have a profoundly unhealthy mind-body-spirit connection and their life will be stunted accordingly.

You have to learn to laugh at yourself and enjoy your life. In addition, as I explain to my patients at our addiction clinic, it's essential to dump your addicted friends. You will never recover from an addiction by keeping these negative influences in your life. To cure drug addiction, an important step is to remove other drug addicts from your environment. In the same way, remove the negative influences in your life, including your negative friends. Life is too short and you have too much to give. Anyone who brings you down will have that effect on your life as well. They are symptoms of a negative spiral that leads to disease.

It's all part of the mind-body-spirit connection that pervades your life. A small, positive change in one area will cause spontaneous improvements in other parts of your life. Before you know it, your life is replete with a sparkling, buoyant wholeness that helps you to look forward with great enthusiasm to every single day.

It's hard to change this sort of thinking overnight. You have to do it in stages. It's a process. There's no such thing as an anti-aging pill, only a steady progression toward better-quality days and greater longevity. As I've said before, the slow, small changes are key; they may not be visible at first, but they will reap long-term dividends.

Before you know it, you are in a cycle of positivity. It takes a little bit of effort, but not a lot. Start small, and you will experience an exponential chain reaction throughout your life that leads to better, more enjoyable days.

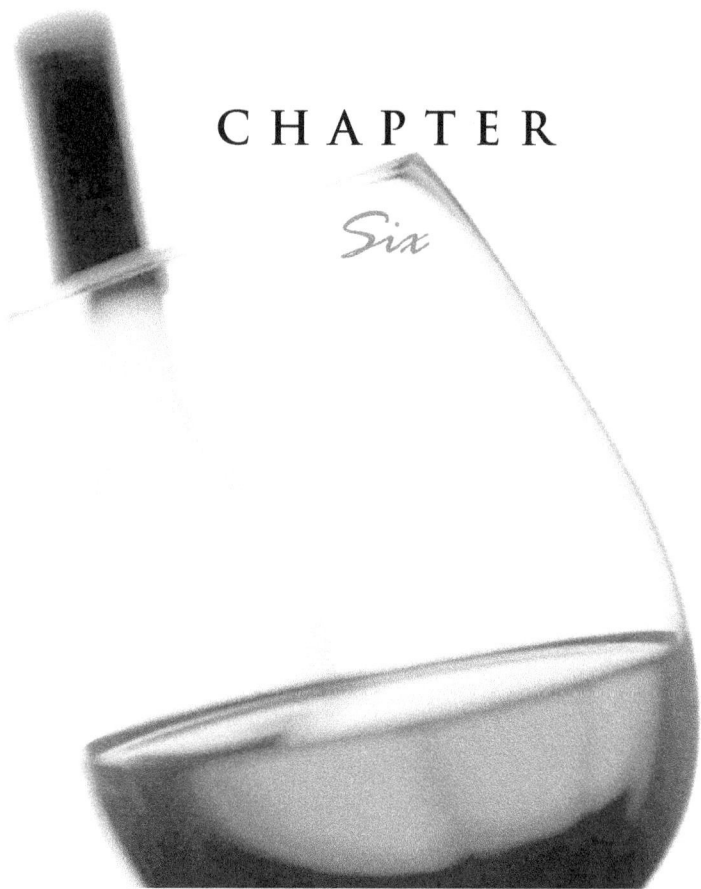

CHAPTER

Six

CHAPTER SIX

Your Body in Motion

"If you rest, you rust."

Helen Hayes

There is no doubt that, as we age, everything slows down. Our hormones decline; physical strength gets challenged; digestion is less efficient; everything just diminishes. That's one reason why I emphasize balancing yourself on all levels; it makes it easier to handle the challenges that aging will bring you.

Combine exercise with a good, nourishing diet and bioidentical hormones; they all work together, ensuring the quality and quantity of your longevity. These three factors are completely interdependent. Moderate exercise staves off disease and ensures strength and flexibility; it depends on good nutrition to provide the fuel that sustains your activity levels. Exercise improves and stabilizes your body's hormones; optimum hormone levels restore your youthful enthusiasm, making you want to get active. Exercise improves your body's metabolism of nutrients; more lean muscle helps you to burn even more calories for a trimmer physique.

If you owned a Ferrari, you would want to put premium gasoline in it, not regular fuel, to ensure that it runs at peak efficiency. Your own premium fuel is a combination of bioidentical hormones, ongoing exercise, and high-quality nutrition; they all work synergistically together. Once you have regained the joy in your life, including good mobility and a high quality of life, everything else will continue to look up. You feel like you can accomplish anything or do anything, and that's tremendously rewarding.

With people who start following this powerful regimen, their demeanor and outlook on life completely changes. This is as satisfying for me to witness, as their doctor, as it is for them to experience it. Exercise is a critical component in this attractive scenario.

Many of the changes that physiologists attribute to aging are actually caused by disuse. Using your body will keep it young; the longer you remain active, the more likely that you will live a long, vigorously healthy life with ample strength and mobility.

Regular aerobic exercise literally slows down the aging process. It floods the body with oxygen to generate energy and enhance overall functioning. It prevents major diseases and injury, speeds recovery, and helps you to get sick less often. It enhances mood and helps you to deal more effectively with stress through the release of endorphins, which also have a natural pain-killing effect.

It can also shave 10 to 12 years off your chronological age, according to various studies. One was published in the *Annals of Internal Medicine;* it studied more than 1000 pairs of twins and compared lifestyle factors. Twins who performed close to 3.5 hours of physical activity per week appeared up to 10 years younger, with less heart disease, cancer, diabetes, hypertension, obesity, and osteoporosis compared to their counterparts.

Trying to hold on to your twenties doesn't make sense. You may want to color your hair and exercise to look good, but you certainly don't want to dress like a 20-year-old. Celebrate your age! Cultivate this attitude because it's an exciting life no matter what age you are.

Like the initial inertia of a stationary object, moving into a healthy active lifestyle may be difficult at first. But getting started is the most difficult step. Soon you'll recapture the glowing vitality and healthy constitution of your youth and you'll never look back. You'll not only look good, you'll feel good, and that is a natural motivator.

Small Changes, Big Reward

The human body is designed to move often, in as many different ways as possible, but modern living seems to thwart this inclination at every turn. We drive everywhere; work primarily at desk jobs; juggle packed schedules that seem to blissfully obstruct our attempts at getting active; and live in concrete jungles that appear to limit our activity options to the same boring roster.

Yet the fact remains that exercise is absolutely crucial to remaining actively, youthfully vigorous. Overcoming the societal obstacles to getting active will take a change in your attitude. Get to work on devising ways to include activity in your day. The choice is up to you.

How do you want to live the rest of your days? Just 30 minutes of brisk, daily walking will enhance your health and reduce your risk for many of the chronic illnesses that cause debilitation in older individuals. It is never too late to start getting active: one Harvard University study showed that nursing-home patients between the ages of 87 and 90 years of age gained muscle, strength, and bone density when involved in a weight-lifting program.

Another study from Israel concluded that previously sedentary people who start to exercise at the age of 85 are twice as likely to be alive, three years later, as people of the same age who remained sedentary. As reported in the *Archives of Internal Medicine*, scientists found that four hours a week of walking was as beneficial as rigorous or prolonged exercise for these older subjects. They also suffered less depression and loneliness and gained a greater ability to perform daily tasks.

The Dallas Bed Rest and Training Study studied a group of men, and then followed up on them 30 years later, to prove that getting active at the age of 50 can produce the same benefits as the workouts of a 20-year-old. At the end of six months of regular exercise, the men averaged a reasonable, 10-pound loss in weight. They also reset their cardiovascular systems very nearly to those recorded when they were 20 years old, including blood pressure, resting heart rate, and the heart's maximum pumping ability. This study concluded that regular exercise had effectively reversed 30 years of decline in their aerobic capacity.

The scientists advocated walking, jogging, and biking for their exercise. Other excellent forms of aerobic activity include swimming, racquet sports, rowing, cross-country skiing, aerobic dance, and even golf (without using an electric cart, of course). The key to ongoing fitness is committing to regular activity. If you are mostly inactive at present, be sure to start slowly. This ensures that being out of shape doesn't lead to an injury that would derail your goal.

Build up gradually to three or four hours of exercise a week. A program as simple as 30 minutes of brisk walking nearly every day will produce major benefits. Enjoying activities with friends is a great way to get motivated; golf, racquet sports, hiking, or dancing are good examples of buddy-friendly exercise.

Pedometers will also help to motivate you by recording how much you walk each day. In a study of 58 inactive women, published in *Medicine & Science in Sports & Exercise,* those who wore a pedometer and aimed for 10,000 steps daily walked farther than those who simply aimed to take a brisk, 30-minute walk per day.

A consistent, ongoing commitment to moving and stretching your body will keep it strong and supple throughout the remainder of your years. But the benefits of exercise extend much farther to positively affect every area of your life.

Fit and Fabulous

There is nothing more motivating for getting active than a trip to the doctor and an ominous test result: high blood pressure, elevated cholesterol, or other similar threat. Many sincere exercise programs have begun out of such fear. However, sticking with your initial commitment can require a different sort of motivation. The following information will develop your understanding of the positive health benefits provided by exercise; hopefully, it will support your desire to remain active.

Exercise protects against such widely disparate conditions as heart disease, colds, dementia, hot flashes, gum disease, stress, diabetes, excess body fat, and depression. It supports your immune system, improves sleep, protects your bones, joints, and vision, and improves wound healing, sex, job performance, and the prospects of career advancement. How many other activities can you name with such wide-reaching benefits?

When it comes to the heart, exercise helps to lower bad cholesterol, raise good cholesterol, improve circulation, repair damaged arteries and keep them flexible, lower blood pressure, and reduce the risk of blood clots. Because exercise helps with so many cardiac risk factors, it is powerfully protective against heart attacks, which are a major killer of mature North Americans. In 1976, the Harvard Alumni Study determined that men who exercised regularly were 39 percent less likely to suffer heart attacks than their sedentary peers. This groundbreaking observation has been confirmed through many subsequent studies.

Stroke, which is the third-leading cause of death in America, is often caused by atherosclerosis. This condition, in which the arteries become clogged and hardened with fatty deposits, is also implicated in heart attacks; it is dramatically improved with exercise. In 2002, the Harvard Alumni Study proved that mild exercise could lead to a 24 percent reduction in the risk of having a stroke; moderate to intensive exercise reduced the risk even further to 46 percent.

Exercise can also help fight the nation's second leading killer: cancer. Colon cancer offers the clearest demonstration of exercise's benefits. Another Harvard study, the Health Professionals Follow-Up Study, found that highly active men are 47 percent less likely to develop the disease than their sedentary peers; this conclusion has been supported through many other studies.

More research shows that keeping active prevents and alleviates depression and stabilizes mood swings. Research into anxiety and depression, reported by the Mayo Clinic (mayoclinic.com), indicates the physical benefits of exercise: the release of "feel-good" chemicals neurotransmitters and endorphins elevates mood while reducing inflammatory responses that can worsen depression.

While all this feel-good physiology is going on, exercise also offers a potent diversion from negative thoughts and worries, which can feed anxiety and depression. As well, being physically active helps to boost self-confidence through meeting fitness goals, overcoming physical challenges, and improving your appearance.

Socially-based activity, such as partner or team sports, helps you to connect with others while fostering that important attachment to community I discussed in chapter 5. It is identified in *The Blue Zones* as an essential ingredient for longevity. Simply exchanging a friendly smile or greeting as you walk around your neighborhood can help you to remain cheerful, which enhances your health.

Doing something salubrious and positive for yourself is a healthy coping strategy. It is a much better choice for managing the stressors in your life than addictive behaviors such as overeating, drinking, or taking hallucinogenic drugs.

Exercise improves blood flow; all that cardiac pumping helps to flush toxins from your lymphatic system. The build-up of years of toxins can be released by taking up a fitness program. Toxins flow out of the body through the blood, and are excreted as waste. This very important process reduces your aches and pains, sharpens your mental acuity, and supports your body in mature health.

The difference between people who will age well and those who won't lies in how fast their minds continue to work. Exercise is also a contributing factor. In addition to increasing the neurotransmitters serotonin, dopamine, and norepinephrine, exercise has been found to increase the levels of brain-derived neurotrophic factor (BDNF). This substance's primary role seems to be in helping brain cells survive longer. A patient's recovery from traumatic brain injury is related in part to the up-regulation of BDNF from exercise.

Studies show that consistent physical activity will help to keep the brain in good shape, reducing the risk of Alzheimer's disease and other dementias. But remember that keeping yourself mentally healthy will also depend on good nutrition and a positive mental attitude.

Weight Management

When you keep your body active and healthy, things begin to happen at the molecular level: your brain starts changing; you become less insulin resistant; and you burn more calories, which helps you to maintain a healthy weight. Exercise reduces your body fat and the overall size of fat cells; it improves your body's use of insulin and lowers blood-sugar levels. Aerobic activity also suppresses your appetite by acting on hormones that regulate hunger.

Muscle burns more calories. The more muscle you have, the more body fat you burn, even while resting. Adding three pounds of muscle will increase your resting metabolic rate by 7 percent while improving your body's ability to utilize protein to sustain and increase muscle. The mitochondria in your muscles produce the energy that keeps you moving, taking fuel from stored fat to keep this process going. If you restrict your calories by 25 percent and combine that with an exercise program, you'll burn 15 percent more calories and will also decrease your aging by 30 percent.

Exercise plays a huge role in improving the insulin resistance I discussed in chapter 4. By adding exercise to your day, you can boost your cellular insulin receptors to about 25,000, which means that you can metabolize more sugar and minimize the danger of insulin resistance. You also use up sugar quickly through exercise, creating a healthful solution to the occasional, unhealthy meal.

Along with hormone-boosting foods, exercise is particularly helpful for low-thyroid conditions (see chapter 3 for more information about supporting your thyroid). Just 20 minutes a day of brisk walking, such as during your lunch hour, will not only increase your circulation but stimulate your thyroid gland. Production of the T4 thyroid hormone is increased by almost 35 percent with exercise; this level will remain high in direct proportion to the length of your workout. Regular, daily activity will keep your T4 levels stable throughout the day to increase metabolic processes and energy levels and improve your mood.

Active and Sexy

Physical fitness determines your ability to function independently and plays a large role in self-esteem. As youth takes its final curtain call, the negative emphasis our culture places on aging can severely erode your confidence with every wrinkle, sag, and bulge. Dissatisfaction with what your mirror shows can affect how you present yourself to the world and how you expect to be treated.

It can also affect your enthusiasm for sex; getting naked was much easier in the days when a youthfully firm body was being uncovered. The desire to keep an out-of-shape figure hidden can quench sexual desire, and sex is one of the best forms of exercise around. Regular exercise improves muscle tone, which also enhances sexual performance.

When you're working out, your creative juices get stimulated and your libido starts increasing. People who begin exercising report an increase in erotic dreams. Slowly and imperceptibly, the quality of your sex life is boosted with continuous activity.

Exercise and Hormones

Exercise also naturally increases and regulates hormone production in your body. For both scxcs, a consistently active lifestyle is a superb complement to bioidentical hormone therapy. If your hormones are out of balance, your body will not respond optimally to improved nutrition and exercise.

With the combined power of bioidentical hormones, consistent exercise, and quality nutrition, every part of you will begin to function like a top-performing orchestra. Your body will hum with the same hormone levels as you had in your youth; your brain will be sharp and focused; your bones will be stronger; your muscles will remain powerful with better overall tone; and you will forever enjoy the independence provided by physical strength and good mobility.

That "runner's high" that comes from elevated endorphin levels simply can't be beat: 30 minutes of exercise can raise this "feel-good" hormone to five times its resting level. It requires a combination of aerobic and strength training. The longer you work out, the more endorphins you will create and the longer they will circulate in your system to sustain those good feelings.

However, studies have shown that exercise can also raise the level of cortisol, especially in mature individuals. Exercise deliberately stresses the body to strengthen it; as I discussed in the previous chapter, stress can result in dangerously high cortisol production. Since too much cortisol can wreak havoc on your beneficial hormones, how then can you exercise safely?

Actually, exercise is one of the best ways to lower cortisol levels because it increases the "feel-good hormones" dopamine and serotonin; endorphin levels are also increased. All this contentment helps to reduce the need for cortisol in response to stress. I recommend consistent, moderate exercise to ensure that your cortisol levels stay under control.

Studies indicate that regular exercise helps to change the body's response to hormones. With cortisol, it trains the body to react more efficiently to increased levels. At least 30 minutes of moderate exercise, four to five times a week, activates this process.

However, too much intensive, excessive exercising can elevate cortisol, especially if your fitness level cannot easily sustain this level. So ensure that you do not over-exercise; a series of intensive workouts lasting more than an hour can cause this to occur in some individuals.

Studies show that taking magnesium after aerobic exercise helps to reduce cortisol levels. In addition, when you realize that you are under excessive stress, you can support your hormone levels by switching to more tranquil exercises, which are proven to lower cortisol levels. Yoga, water aerobics, stretching exercises, and Tai Chi are good examples.

For women, lifestyle is the most important factor in causing estrogen and progesterone imbalances. Women who eat wholesome food and remain fit have a far lower incidence of menopausal symptoms. This is because their pre- and post-menopause levels of estrogen do not drop as significantly. Regular exercise has a normalizing effect on estrogen levels, improving the crucial estrogen-to-progesterone ratio.

Another very beneficial hormone, DHEA, will naturally increase with exercise. The production of this "master hormone" offers tremendous health benefits throughout the body (read chapter 3 for more information). For example, it helps to combat adrenal fatigue, supports the healthy functioning of the adrenal glands, and is instrumental in the creation of the sex hormones.

Of particular note, increasing DHEA through supplementation or via exercise can elevate testosterone levels in both sexes, which in turn can benefit muscles, bones, concentration, and libido. Exercise is the best way to enhance testosterone, which will help to maintain or build muscle and increase stamina and strength. Testosterone also boosts metabolism, making your body use food more efficiently and burn fat faster.

As a man ages, declining testosterone levels are linked to the loss of muscle. This can reduce a man's musculature by up to 50 percent in later years. Healthy testosterone levels from regular exercise help to prevent this condition of weakness and disability. They also provide an important basis of support for a man's libido, and studies have linked regular exercise to a 30 percent reduction in a man's risk of impotence.

Any package of intervention must include regular exercise at its core.

In addition, while men have a lower risk of osteoporosis than women, they do lose bone calcium with age, which increases the risk of fractures.

A drop in testosterone may be so significant in some men that they have none to spare to aromatize into estrogen. As we learned in chapter 3, men require a minimum amount of estrogen to prevent osteoporosis and bone fractures. This combination of low testosterone and low estrogen levels will lead to higher mortality without intervention. Any package of intervention must include regular exercise at its core to help increase and maintain good testosterone levels. It is important for protecting a man's mature constitution on all levels.

Kester's Core

For both sexes, exercise improves hormone functions, and getting active is a key factor in aging to perfection. Bioidentical hormone therapy supports this process by enhancing your overall well-being. It ensures that you benefit from optimum hormone levels as you pursue a vigorous, active lifestyle.

For people who have always enjoyed a potent, robust activity level, bioidentical hormone therapy can play an important role in protecting their athletic performance. The following story illustrates how this therapy worked to restore the performance of a lifelong athlete.

Kester Jackson had always been very active, enjoying all types of outdoor activities. "I have always been concerned about my physical well-being, whether for play or my very active career in business development," he says. If you were to see a photo of this high achiever, you would never believe that he was in his sixties. He is a poster child for the tremendous benefits that come from remaining physically active.

While in his thirties, he became involved in competitive power lifting, which he enjoyed tremendously until his early sixties; he then noticed a considerable drop in his performance. "My ability to recover from strenuous exercise started waning." Numerous orthopedic issues with his shoulder and knee joints led to seven operations, along with arthritis, which further sapped his strength and confidence. His surgeon told him about bioidentical hormone therapy and how it could assist him, and Kester came to me for an assessment.

I did a thorough physical, including taking his health history and doing blood work, then recommended he begin therapy with bioidentical testosterone. We chose pellet therapy, inserted under the skin, and I also recommended some nutraceutical supplements to balance his body's functioning, including Alpha Lipoic Acid, Co-enzyme Q10, and DHEA.

After the first pellet was inserted, I monitored how it was working in his body with three sets of blood tests and inserted a second pellet four months later. Kester was delighted with the effects of this therapy. "The difference has been very dramatic. My strength has increased back to levels that I was capable of when I was in my forties. My overall feeling of well-being is excellent and my libido has come back to levels I had in my early years. My mind seems to be sharper than ever and my recovery time from workouts is fantastic," he says.

"I train cardio every day of the week, for forty minutes, and train core and weight training three to four days a week. I have leaned out through my mid-section again and my abdominal definition is back to what it was in my thirties," he says. Kester's excellent physical condition provided tremendous benefits in helping him retain his youthful strength and vitality. He has always known that fitness was an important component in achieving his goals of personal and professional success. It has given him the stamina and energy to get everything he desires out of his life.

However, even for a fitness buff, the quality of his life was beginning to suffer. This natural athlete was being affected by the slow decline in testosterone that comes with maturity. It affects us all, until we choose to stop it from happening. Hormone imbalance of any kind can sap one's physical prowess and stamina. Perhaps the most devastating effect is a loss of confidence in how your own body functions.

The relentless march of aging was insidiously affecting his well-being, physical strength, mental clarity, and sex life. It may have been his ongoing commitment to exercise that helped him to pinpoint the changes that often go unnoticed in a man because they happen so slowly (testosterone levels decline at a rate of one to two percent per year; see chapter 3 for more details).

Bioidentical hormone therapy and the strategic use of nutraceuticals helped to repair what nature was destroying. Getting his body back into balance allowed Kester to resume bench-pressing and free-weight-squats at around 300 pounds each. "It really kick-started my training into the next level within four months," he says. "I plan to continue this regimen for many years to come."

Kester also expressed appreciation for the sympathetic and supportive approach that is part of functional medicine: a personalized treatment paradigm focused on resolving the underlying causes of disease. "I am very pleased with the results that Dr. Garcia has been able to achieve with his well-conceived anti-aging program."

Get Out There

By now, I hope that you are convinced: getting out there and getting active is worth the commitment. You can look forward to all the benefits that you are about to experience. So here are some myths, common to exercise, that I would like to dispel to further encourage you.

To get more active, you have to change your whole life. Not so, say experts. Studies show that 10-minute bouts of any type of aerobic activity, two or more times a day, will produce significant benefits.

There is not enough time in the day. I realize that we are a time-strapped culture, but Americans still find the time to watch $4\frac{1}{2}$ hours of television per day. If this is you, then you have enough time to exercise. At the very least, get active during commercial breaks instead of getting a snack. Or you can exercise during your lunch hour. You can also go for your workout before you begin your workday; this is actually the best time because few people can find the time after work.

Exercise is boring. Remember that any type of movement counts as exercise, and there is a lot of potential movement out there. You can enjoy an evening of square dancing, which is comparable to walking five miles. Ballroom dancing can burn more calories than gym-style aerobics. Think beyond walking, jogging, or structured routines; vary your choices as much as you can to make being active endlessly enjoyable.

You can also include family members and friends and take active vacations: you can get in a lot of walking while enjoying Disney World with your children. Whatever you do, such as hiking in the Smoky Mountains of Colorado or wilderness camping, these kinds of vacations can form lasting bonds and create lifelong memories as well as increase the fitness level of all participants.

Exercise will make you eat more. In fact, the reverse is true. Studies show that exercise suppresses the appetite. In 2008, a study of 15 obese men and women was presented at the Endocrine Society's 90th Annual meeting in San Francisco. Three months of regular exercise on a treadmill or bicycle was shown to actually reduce appetite, even though participants were told not to change their eating habits.

You have to wear special clothes and sweat. Okay, this is true for some sports but many activities simply require comfortable clothing. One example is Tai Chi, an ancient Chinese martial art, which consists of deep breathing and gentle, slow, controlled movements. Tai Chi improves blood sugar in diabetics, relieves stress, and enhances heart and lung health, the immune system, and overall flexibility, all without having to shed a single drop of sweat.

Exercise is exhausting. If this is true, then you're going at it too hard; exercise actually improves endurance rather than detracting from it. The trick here is to start slow, especially if you have been sedentary for a long time. Be consistent and your energy levels will increase. Start with gentle stretches, first thing in the morning. After a few days, go for a walk after stretching and then stretch again afterwards.

It is best to start very slowly; for example, begin by walking for five minutes a day, and then increasing to ten minutes, and gradually working up to thirty minutes on most days. Walk your dog; walk in the morning with a friend; or join a walking club. Walk briskly enough to breathe more heavily than usual, but still be able to talk. Getting active will take a little bit of initiative and perseverance. But if you're reading this book, you are already motivated to change. And once you start walking around the block, it creates such tremendous dividends that you are motivated to do more.

You have to join a gym. There are thousands of workout DVDs to choose from and many cable-television channels dedicated to fitness. Another option is the Wii Fit (WiiFit.com), a game-style program that connects to your television to provide personal training tailored to your own preference and fitness level; it is also fun.

Exercise will hurt aching or stiff joints. Again, this is contrary to popular belief. Exercise is a natural pain reliever because it causes the release of endorphins. A recent study of 346 people with arthritis published in the American College of Rheumatology's online *Arthritis Care and Research Journal* (interscience.wiley.com) found that one hour of low-impact exercise, twice a week, reduced pain and fatigue and improved joint function.

Walking is all you ever need to do. This is true if you've been sedentary for a long time; walking does produce significant health benefits. But one of the realities of fitness is that, as you do more exercise, your fitness level increases. You have to challenge your muscles to continue improving and you will eventually require more intense aerobic and resistance exercise to produce benefits. An exercise program should become more challenging, not stay static, unless you're not doing it regularly. You need to continually improve your heart and muscles to improve your fitness.

It is impossible to get motivated. Many times I have seen people who do not get started with a good diet or exercise regime until they are faced with a major health crisis. At this point they're finally motivated enough to do something about their health. Although they will still benefit, this stage is somewhat late and tremendous damage may have already been done.

Don't let this be you! Whatever it takes, such as hiring a coach, begging a buddy, or investing your hard-earned money and time, just do it. Make your health a priority and your life will be prioritized accordingly. It won't kill you to get more active. But not doing so will eventually kill you.

Go to the library and read up on activities that might interest you. Choose a few of them, and then bring a positive mindset to your intention to exercise. Set some goals each week, and then work toward reaching them. Share those goals with a friend or loved one and ask them to monitor, encourage, or browbeat you into achieving them. Plan some incentives to keep yourself going: a new piece of equipment, going away for an active weekend, or other financial reward.

Commit to doing whatever it takes to get active. The rest of your life depends on it.

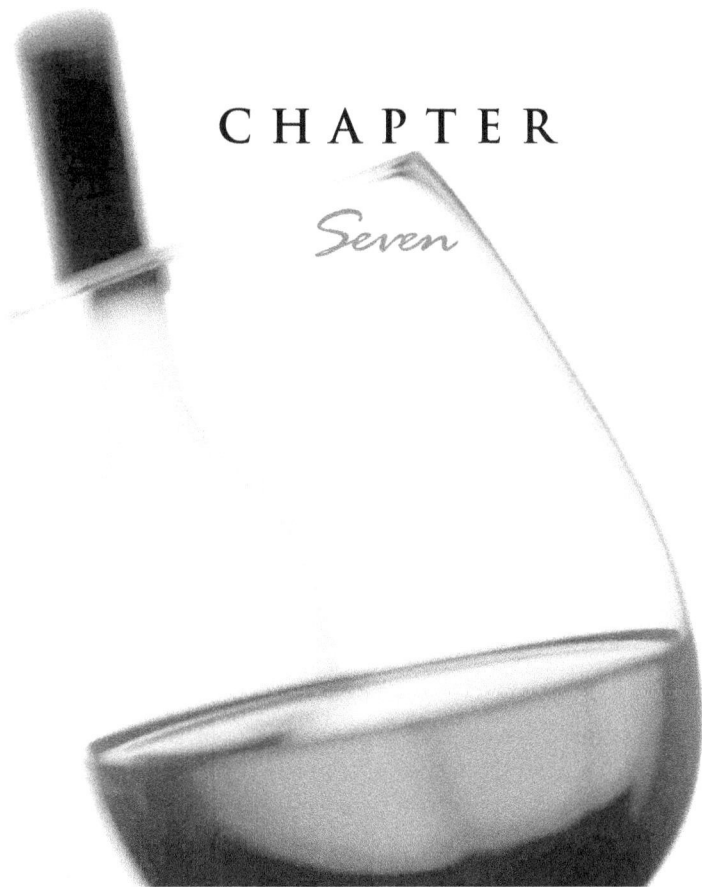

CHAPTER

Seven

CHAPTER SEVEN

Your Mind and Spirit Shape Your Body

"Your beliefs become your thoughts.
Your thoughts become your words.
Your words become your actions.
Your actions become your habits.
Your habits become your values.
Your values become your destiny."

Mahatma Gandhi

Your attitude, which is so important to your success in reversing age-related conditions, is an expression of your mind and spirit and has a profound effect on what happens to your body. On the journey back to greater energy and flawless health, everyone is coming from a different place, but the body-mind-spirit connection is always involved.

In previous chapters, I discussed how the quality of your mature life is affected by your body-mind-spirit connection. All that you currently are, and all that you hope to become, depends on this connection. For example, your mental understanding of age-related conditions gives you the knowledge to make healthier choices. But your ability to regain your health doesn't exist in this knowledge; the key is your attitude, or willingness, to make the small and incremental lifestyle changes based on this knowledge.

This book has equipped you with an understanding of the healthy foods and nutraceuticals that will help to maintain a glowing constitution. While they comprise the physical act of keeping healthy, the attitude you bring to nourishing yourself will determine your success in this challenge. The same goes for exercise and the way in which you respond physically to stress.

Traumatized Genes

Environmental factors including past experiences appear to influence the expression of both your stress and longevity genes. This is seen in studies involving identical twins who have the same genes yet differ in appearance, lifespan, and health. Epigenetics, which literally means "control above the genes," is the study of gene expression caused by mechanisms other than changes in the underlying DNA. It is an emerging science that explores how environmental factors express or suppress an inherited genetic trait.

There is a clear connection between the experience of deep trauma and the development of diseases. Studies indicate that children who are not nurtured in early life have a much higher incidence of disease. Part of the reason is that children who are not nurtured lose their ability to handle stress. They have five times the chance of being depressed, are three times as likely to smoke, and are thirty times more likely to attempt suicide. Those who grew up in dysfunctional families were more likely to suffer from obesity, heart disease, lung disease, diabetes, bone fractures, hypertension, or hepatitis.

Researchers found that the more traumatic the childhood, the higher the disease risk. It's the mind-body connection being expressed; there is something happening at the cellular level. Epigenetic research suggests that the subconscious mind can be affected to such a point that it turns on "stress genes," leading to a cascade of hormonal events that results in disease (see chapter 5 for more information about the stress response).

Genes are turned on by different experiences. For example, we know through advanced DNA microarray technology ("gene scans") that lonely and depressed people turn on 200 separate sets of gene switches. These scans help us to determine what genes are activated by what mechanisms. It was once thought that our genes controlled our characteristics in a one-to-one direct relationship (the "Central Dogma" of genetics, where one gene makes one protein), but now we know that there are three million different expressions of our 23,688 genes.

They are expressed through the foods we eat (unhealthy foods will lead to the expression of diseases, and vice versa) and through our experiences (positive ones express good genes and unresolved traumas will lead to the expression of disease). Even thoughts and feelings turn sets of genes on and off, unleashing a particular cascade of biochemicals in our organs from moment to moment; each experience triggers genetic changes in our cells.

The molecules of our emotions are inseparable from our physiology because they help to determine our physiology. What this means is that you are not predestined to live and die exactly as your parents did. You can overcome your genetic inheritance, over which you had no control, by effecting the good expression of genes through factors that you do control, such as modifying your diet, behavior, or attitudes. This is the body-mind-spirit connection at play.

An example of this can be found in a recent study where switching to a healthy lifestyle, including an improved diet (rich in whole grains, fruits, legumes, soy, and vegetables), moderate exercise (walking), and reduced stress (an hour a day spent in a stress-reduction activity such as meditation) showed measurable results within three months. It increased telomerase and was beneficial in controlling the aging process. Telomerase is an enzyme that maintains the length of the telomere, a region at the tip of a cell's chromosome that determines its lifespan. After each cell division, the telomere diminishes to the point that, at a certain length, the cell is unable to divide further and will undergo senescence (it dies). This is called the Hayflick Limit. It is believed that maintaining a longer telomere by activation of telomerase may contribute to a longer life by preventing cell senescence.

The researchers in this study found that men achieved a 29 percent higher level of telomerase through the introduction of simple lifestyle interventions. They were able to use gene scans to see which genes were switched off or on. They found an epigenetic effect on 501 genes (48 genes were turned on and 453 genes were turned off) based solely on the positive lifestyle changes these men had made.

Mind the Brain

The brain is something we see, whereas the mind is what we don't see. The brain is your body's "command center." It controls your basic, physiological functions of movement, thoughts, and emotions. Neurotransmitters and hormones are the language your brain uses to direct your body's functions. The mind is the emotional center, the "unconscious genius" and effectively the person's soul. You can look at yourself apart from your physical brain, and that is your mind and your soul.

Your brain controls all of your physiological responses and your mind reacts to stimuli and dictates what the brain will do. The two are linked, but their functions are very different. For example, with any kind of stress, your mind will perceive the stressor and then relate to it via certain ingrained behaviors or expectations; then your brain will initiate certain chemical or hormonal responses.

The actual stress response is your brain, but the perception of stress is your mind. Your childhood traumas are mostly subconscious and yet they are physically expressed, for example as a hyper-reaction to a threat. This excessive "stress response" can be controlled with techniques designed to change your subconscious response. These include guided imagery, relaxation training, deep breathing, and meditation.

Strong emotional experiences create immunological changes in the body. If you have vowed revenge against someone, this creates a stress response in your body that will ultimately increase the amount of cortisol, triggering an inflammatory cascade that will eventually lead to the expression of disease unless you can let go of that negativity and learn to forgive.

You have to release resentments because this early conditioning toward negative reactions will create disease later in life. It's not a one-way street; you can reverse it. Your disease genes were activated by your early experiences and you can turn them off again by developing the ability to react differently. This is the divine healing process at work in which healing the body first requires healing the spirit. Through counseling, or developing positive mental attitudes centered around learning to love life, your whole attitude can change and then different genes will kick in to reverse the pattern of disease.

The cycle of positivity, the need for positive outlook, or what I call the merry heart, takes a little bit of effort to achieve. It comes down to that classic question: Is the glass half full or half empty? You can change your whole being and your whole health by changing your attitude. But you have to change it.

Some people are caught in neutral; they're stuck in the mud and refuse to give it up. They won't forgive anybody and won't let go of their anger; they won't give up their resentments and let go of whatever happened. They will pay the price with chronic disease and an early death.

Laughter and Fear

Laughter is perhaps the best medicine by all accounts for dealing with chronic stress, which can devastate the immune system. Laughter actually alters your body's physical response to stress, including emotional and environmental stress. With enough laughter and the right nutrition, you can enhance your body's response to virtually any health challenge.

Studies show that laughter will help you to heal injuries more quickly, recover from surgery faster, fight infection more effectively, reduce your perception of pain, alleviate or eliminate symptoms of depression, and just feel better about being alive. Laughter helps you take yourself and your life less seriously. It connects your mind and body together through a "merry heart."

Fear creates the same connection with devastating results. Consider the following two cases: a man died of cancer, yet the autopsy showed that there weren't enough spots of cancer in his body to have killed him. A priest administered the last rights to the wrong patient, and then the patient died unexpectedly. These are two examples of how fear caused disease and even death.

This ancient concept was formalized decades ago by Dr. Robert K. Meton; he defined this as self-fulfilling prophecy. Another term, the "nocebo phenomenon," has been in use since 1961 to describe the reverse placebo effect, where a patient will become sicker after being told of negative side effects, or after being informed of specifics about an illness just diagnosed.

In one experiment, 66 percent of volunteers complained of headaches after being told that an electric current was applied to their heads. In actuality, no current had really been applied. In another study, women holding the belief that they were prone to heart disease died at four times the average rate compared to those who didn't hold such a belief, even though they all started out with the same risk factors.

Preventing age-related disease or declines in healthy vitality is fundamentally dependent on the body-mind-spirit connection. It has been documented that people who believe their memories are soon to fail will actually undergo memory problems earlier than people who may be in similar condition without holding this belief.

In cultures where elderly members are valued highly, mental ability does not deteriorate until much later, if at all, compared to societies where people are dismissed as elderly at the age of 65. In addition, people who are isolated in an environment where growing old is viewed as a disease, such as residents of an assisted-living facility, will age faster than those who live in a mixed-age community where they are not expected to act differently just because they are getting older.

In his book, *The Biology of Belief,* cell biologist Bruce H. Lipton, PhD, presented compelling evidence that biochemical mechanisms facilitate the phenomenon of mind over matter. Lipton challenged traditional cell theory, which basically defines cells as inflexible, closed units programmed to do only one job; instead, he says, cells are like blank computer chips waiting to be programmed to take on different jobs.

The former Stanford professor says that a cell is built to act on its own in an isolated environment such as a laboratory, but when it becomes part of a community it subjugates this individuality. All the cells then receive collective programming instructions from the life force, such as a person. As messages are sent to the cell for action, it is the information-receiving process that determines the cell's behavior, not some built-in, fixed programming.

Simply stated, this means that there is no cancer gene. Illness is not inherited. Rather, cells become cancerous because they were told to do so. Fear can drive such instruction. The good news is that the mind-body relationship can also work in reverse and a positive attitude is a prime factor in the health you will enjoy.

Your Brain's Power

There is a clear connection between exercise and brain power. Exercise gives more creativity to your work. I'm always amazed, when I am running on my treadmill, at what pops into my brain that I have never considered before. Part of the reason is serotonin, the "feel-good" hormone that greatly contributes to an overall sense of well-being. It also helps to regulate moods, temper anxiety, and relieve depression.

In addition, what you eat is very intimately connected to how you think. The brain is 70 percent fat and this is what it needs to function optimally. But I'm not talking about fried foods and trans fats. You need to eat good fats, such as omega-3 oils: fish oils, flax seed oil, and olive oil; all these help the brain to work at peak efficiency.

To improve the functioning of your mind, reduce depression, and support your mood, you also need nutritious, whole foods such as a plant-based diet of organic food. From epigenetics we know that the food you eat will affect the expression of genetic traits. I've always said that bad food expresses disease genes and good food equates to health because health genes are expressed.

Can nutrition overwhelm depression? It can, in many ways. An alert mind and a sense of well-being are enhanced by proper nutrition and certain nutraceutical supplements. It just makes everything work better.

Supplements are good, and I am on them myself, but you also need nutritious, whole foods. Nature, in its wisdom, has created the ideal combination of minerals, vitamins, and enzymes in each plant, offering the maximum nutritional benefit. The whole makeup of the plant is healthy. You can put a picture of a plant on a bottle but it doesn't mean that you will have the same nutritional benefit from taking that pill as you will from eating a whole food.

However, for people who are not eating right or not exercising, a little supplementation with nutraceuticals can help them to overcome nutritional deficiencies. Within 30 days, they start feeling better and are more able to follow a healthy program of nutrition, exercise, and positive attitudes.

Brain Hormones

The difference between people who are aging to perfection and those who are simply declining into illness and old age is how fast their minds work. Supplementing with bioidentical hormones means that everything works better for a better quality of life. You will be functioning with the same quantity of hormones that you had as a younger person.

For men, our brain hormone is testosterone: it creates more blood flow in every part of the body, including the brain. This aids in functioning and in flushing out toxins. Bioidentical hormone supplementation in mature men is extremely important for healthy functioning, and I'm not talking about the middle range. You have to be in the upper third of the optimal range for testosterone to make a man feel alive, with optimal quality of health, and the ability to function the way he was meant to. Again, as with most laboratory ranges for hormones, the action is in the middle (for more information about this, see chapter 3). Optimization is the key, which means keeping hormone levels in the upper third of the range.

In a similar way, estrogen is important for women, especially during post-menopause. Studies show that it helps a woman's brain to be chemically efficient so that she can think more clearly, with better verbal recall of information. It is part of the brain's signaling system; estrogen helps to direct blood to parts of the brain that are more active. Studies have found that supplementing with bioidentical estrogen reduces the tendency toward memory problems after menopause.

The absence of estrogen is also implicated in the development of macular degeneration in women who enter menopause at a young age. This is why blocking estrogens with the anti-cancer drug tampoxifen is harmful to the retina.

In addition, progesterone stabilizes a woman's moods; it's important for anxiety, depression, and the ability to sleep. After menopause, a woman's progesterone level goes way down and this calming effect is lost, leading to irritability, outbursts of anger, and mood swings. I've seen a lot of women who come to the emergency room complaining of a racing heart, panic attacks, and palpitations, where the common denominator is decreasing progesterone levels.

These women are on antidepressants and anti-anxiety medications because they have been placed in the "it's all in her head" category by a doctor who missed the connection. Bioidentical progesterone reverses this trend for a calmer, more stable mood and an enhanced ability to sleep.

Supporting the thyroid is also very important for a woman's mental health. A lot of women will appear lethargic when they are actually suffering a deficiency in their thyroid hormones. They present with symptoms such as weight gain and feeling cold, but what may not be as readily apparent is their mental deterioration. This includes diminished focus and concentration and an inability to multitask the way they used to. They know that something is wrong; they forget their keys, whether they left the stove on, and what they have to shop for, and they feel as though they're losing it, which affects their self-confidence.

People who are on bioidentical hormone supplementation but then go off it will re-experience the original declines in their mental functioning. Once the supplementation is resumed, the improvements return. It's that direct a connection.

Along with stronger bones and muscles, exuberant energy, a robust constitution, and greater mobility, your mind also works better when your hormone levels are optimal. Your brain remains sharply alert and your memory is unimpaired. People who protect their hormone levels with bioidentical supplementation and healthy living practices will protect the quality of their life throughout their mature years.

Improved in Body, Mind, and Spirit

Bioidentical testosterone, along with a healthy diet and nutraceuticals, helped Jason Washington to overcome a lackluster, depressive state of mind stemming from not feeling well. Involved in athletics all of his life, at the age of 44 this African-American man was not recovering from his workouts as easily as he used to. "Over the past few years, I had noticed that my energy level was decreasing, I was more injury prone and just generally feeling lackluster," he recalls.

Jason was still a fit guy and exercised a lot, but it wasn't working for him anymore. He knew something was missing. Then his cholesterol soared to 260. The decline in his health was proving tough to deal with, and Jason was getting discouraged.

He says the most significant sign that something was wrong was in the evening. "I would be so tired I could not stay awake if I tried. There had been times when I would fall asleep midsentence." Depressed about the fact that he was not feeling well, he started having trouble sleeping and also experienced some stress at work.

Researching bioidentical hormone therapy for a friend, he quickly realized this could be a solution for him as well. Then the buddy system kicked in to offer support and validate his research. "Another friend from the gym made the same recommendation. After he informed me of his positive experience, I decided to check it out for myself."

Sometimes the most important thing a doctor can do is offer support and hope. This inspired Jason mentally and spiritually. "Upon my first visit, I knew I was in the right place. Dr. Garcia spent more time with me and was more informative about my health than my regular physician. I left the office with a new plan for eating, vitamin supplements, and bioidentical testosterone replacement."

It took about two months, but he began feeling a lot better. The body-mind-spirit connection is so intertwined that it's difficult to say what improved first: his physical health or his mental stress. It's all interconnected. But he started feeling like a new person. "Within three months, I had lost over ten pounds, maintained muscle, lowered my cholesterol to under 200, and can make it through an entire movie without falling asleep," he says.

External Influences Internal

The brain is an organ that can deteriorate or appreciate, depending on the stimulation you give it. It is exceedingly complex, as it has about 100 billion nerve cells and more connections in it than there are stars in the universe. If you are alone and lonely, or depressed, you end up in a dark place and the mind closes off. After a while, you start to lose brain cells (about 85,000 a day) and synapses (the specialized connectors through which the brain's billions of nerve cells communicate). That's why you need to interact with people, such as socializing and learning new hobbies in addition to regular exercise.

The brain's synaptic connections will continue to develop, even in elderly people. We know that you can continue to build these connections through neuroplasticity, which involves changes to the brain's neurons and the organization of neural networks and functions as a result of new experiences. This is what prevents the onset of Alzheimer's and other dementias.

To some extent, genetics plays a factor in the density of neurons within your brain, but this is only 25 percent of the picture. The rest is entirely up to you. By playing cards or doing word games and puzzles, you stimulate the brain to create new synaptic connections between the neurons and cells. It allows you to think, and remember things, more quickly.

As we age, our thought processes slow down somewhat; we're talking milliseconds here, but it can make a big difference in some people. If you continue to be physically active, with a nutritious diet, it will help to enhance mental functioning.

In addition, the stimulation of interacting with other people enhances neuroplasticity. We know from the cultures profiled in the book *The Blue Zones* that people who live past the age of 100 have in common an attachment to community and good relationships with others. They regularly get together with friends to talk about their lives and community members. It's that interaction with other people that is important: the laughter and connections that are stimulating emotionally but also develop more brain synapses.

I see unhappy elderly people all the time; you learn something from the CAT scans of their heads. They all have atrophy, or shrinking, of the brain. An 80-year-old brain will shrink from sheer age, compared to a 20-year-old brain, but if you can continue stimulating that brain, the decline is less. People who remain active, physically and mentally, are actually protecting their brain power.

In addition, as I discussed in chapter 5, people will develop Alzheimer's and other dementias much faster when they are under stress. This can include feeling lonely or isolated as well as not exercising or eating properly, which are all common challenges for older individuals. Studies show that unremitting stress will eventually shrink the hippocampus; such atrophy has been seen in the brains of patients with dementia, depression, or post-traumatic stress disorder. This shrinkage is also accompanied by memory deficits that arise before atrophy and neuron loss occurs. All facets of your body-mind-spirit connection must be applied toward preventing this frighteningly debilitating condition.

Physically, you must follow a nutritious diet, support the hormonal functioning in your body, and remain active. Mentally, you must continue stimulating the growth of new synapses with "brain training," or constantly using your mental abilities. Spiritually, the development of ongoing, stimulating connections with other people in your community, and faith-based practices, will support both your mood and your mental acuity. You have to balance of all these to protect the quality of your life for the rest of your life.

Healthy Thinking

With all patients, I try to incorporate not just the physical, but the mental and spiritual aspects of health. The way you think has to be dealt with and that may be more difficult than physical challenges because some people just don't get it. Maybe it's too esoteric.

We live in a "pill for every ailment" culture, which is a quick-fix solution without any personal responsibility for taking care of our own health. Many of us think, "If I just take a pill, I will be fine; my doctor will take care of me." But we all have to take the "health bull" by the horns and try to help ourselves as much as possible.

With regard to our own mental health, this requires developing a positive attitude about life. It includes taking regular vacations to completely de-stress. It means addressing unresolved emotional issues you may have, such as with family members and colleagues, so that you will be free to function without the mental stress from such serious hindrances (all stress leads to illness, including mental stress). It means living a more balanced lifestyle.

I've said to people before, "Listen, your job is killing you. You have to make a decision. Do you want to live or do you want to die in your job?" Working long hours is incredibly stressful to your body-mind-spirit connection. As Billy Ray Cyrus once sang, "No one has ever said on their death bed, 'I wish I had spent more time at the office.'"

A mother says to her child, "Do what you love and not what you have to do," and that's not bad advice. What quality of life is possible if you don't love what you are doing? I considered taking up law full-time at one point, but then talked to some lawyers and I swear there is no lawyer who loves his job. They all want to get out. While yearning for something different from what you have is not a healthy attitude, you can find ways to enjoy your life more and minimize the effect of a career that hasn't delivered what it promised.

The grass will always look greener on the other side, and yearning for something else may lead down the path of discontent. But you can look internally, not externally, for your satisfaction; look into yourself, and don't judge what you are doing or feeling by another person's criteria. Use your own, and honestly learn what it is that makes you happy. Then follow it.

If it is necessary for financial reasons to stay in the career you have, then do what you love on a part-time basis. If you want to read, paint, write a book, or do anything else that really turns you on, that's the way to maintain your mental health. Choose a goal that you are passionate about, and then take steps to achieve it. This has tremendous physical and mental benefits. It is much healthier for you than simply watching TV every evening.

What I am talking about is creating an epigenetic self-nurturing environment to surround yourself with, allowing you to better deal with stress, create inner peace, and release your emotional events. Acquiring new skills as an adult that trigger this self-nurturing will pay dividends for your longevity by switching on the genes that promote cell health and reduce inflammation.

It can reverse the negative epigenetic signals that you may have received early on in life through a traumatic childhood. These skills are easy to learn and most of them are free. They include: meditation, prayer, optimism, a positive attitude, energy medicine (reiki, quantum touch, and therapeutic touch), energy psychology (emotional freedom technique), positive beliefs and positive visualizations, acts of kindness and love, and spirituality.

Learning and practicing these skills of self-nurturing can become a catalyst for rekindling the optimism for life that you may have lost long ago.

What Inspires You?

The mind, body, and spirit interact together to enhance or destroy a person's health. Life is not just about physically moving through your days; having a passion for what you do is tremendously motivating and will have a positive impact on your longevity.

The attitude you bring to improving the quality of your life and health will play an important part in whether you will truly change. If you actively work to bring interest and enthusiasm to your daily exercise, nutrition goals, and mental health, and don't make it feel like drudgery, then you will increase your chances for success.

Somehow you have to reach a point where you are going to love it. Otherwise, you will never change your life patterns. Do whatever it takes. Many people are inspired by a partner or companion as they undergo the necessary evolution to a more wholesome, healthful lifestyle. For example, it can be very tough to go for long walks by yourself but fun to explore your community with a partner or friend who can share the fitness journey with you.

It helps to connect with other people as you share your successes and failures. We see that all the time with guys at the gym: one doesn't want to go, but the others say "Let's go, we're going to do it" and they do. The group effort carries the reluctant one along.

You have to vary your activity to enjoy it. The whole purpose of doing different types of physical activity is so that it does not become monotonous drudgery and something that you really hate. If you loathe it, you will not keep at it for very long. Then, as the pounds fall off and your mood improves, you'll become inspired; that is what makes people want to keep going.

People have turned their lives around because I, or someone they love and respect, told them to do something. It's the value of that kind of advice and leadership. They may know it intrinsically, but sometimes hearing it has a tremendous impact.

That's why a mother will bring her three-year-old to the emergency room with a temperature of 103 degrees and vomiting. I know the child's just having a bout of gastroenteritis and it will go away in a few days. But she wants to hear from the doctor that everything is going to be all right. She wants to hear that her child looks good, and is nothing like a child that is truly ill, nothing like a meningitis child, for example. And that relieves her mind to the point where she is grateful. I've seen that so often; sometimes it just has to be said.

The mind controls the body, and a compassionate, sympathetic person can really inspire you. How he turns a word and how he communicates with you has a way of improving your outlook even though you may be dealing with some big challenges.

That's what happens with the placebo effect. In scientific studies, about 30 percent of people who aren't taking the real drug, who are actually taking a placebo or "sugar pill" will still improve because of what the doctor says. This led to double-blind medication studies where neither the subject nor the person giving the drug knows which one is real and which is the placebo. This way, the person running the study (who effectively is in a position of authority) won't unconsciously influence the results with a look, word, or gesture. People are highly susceptible to this kind of influence.

Be inspired by remembering that you're worth it: you are the most valuable creature in the universe to your loved ones. You are! The Earth and the heavens were created for one purpose: you. You have so many things to be thankful and grateful for. Look at all that you have! Remember, gratitude positively affects your attitude.

One patient I've seen in my practice was extremely down and out, as he was depressed by all kinds of superficial things. He's not alone; as human beings, we tend to dwell on the minutiae and disregard the important things around us. Just look around: the magic and majesty of life surrounds you. Change your viewpoint and get inspired by life.

The most beautiful things in the world are free. If you have children, see them as the blessings they are in your life. I've seen the other side: death and dying up close and personal. If you think that you have a bad life, come with me for a tour of the cancer ward at the Children's Hospital of Columbus, Ohio. You will come out of your depression in a microsecond because that is real pain.

One of my doctor friends in the emergency room took up playing tennis, and now she flies to the Australian Open each January. Her passion for her sport inspired its own momentum. She wants to watch professional tennis; her husband started going with her and now it has become an adventure, as well as a journey. The excitement builds, they have mementos from all these places they've visited, they've met many interesting and exciting people from other cultures, and their conversation at the dinner table with family and friends includes much from their travels. Her exercise goal has expanded to enhance her life in so many ways. You don't necessarily have to be that expansive, but I think the same kind of thing happens on a smaller scale with many people who find inspiring ways to reach their goal.

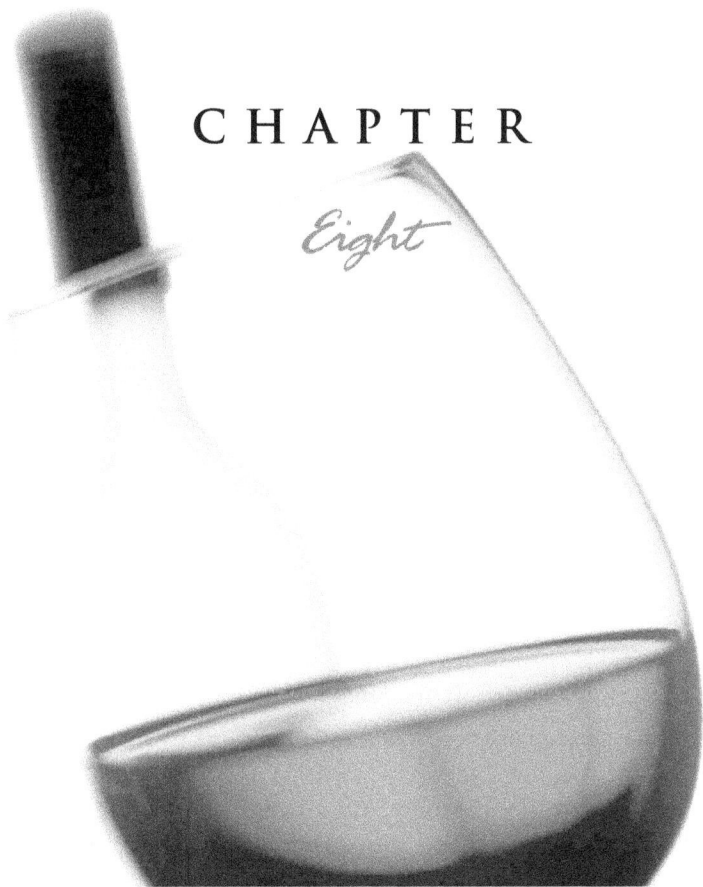

CHAPTER

Eight

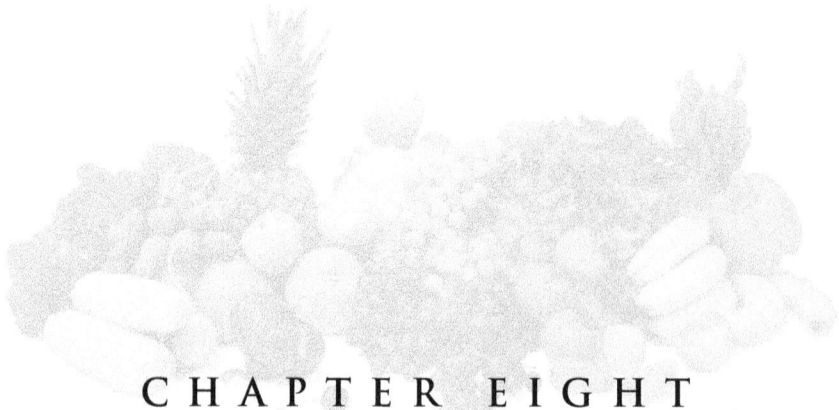

CHAPTER EIGHT

Awareness of Your Environment

"At the end of times the merchants of the world will deceive the nations through their Pharmacia." (Sorcery)

R e v .   1 8 : 2 3

How prevalent are environmental toxins in our modern lives? Consider the following typical, daily routine and my subsequent scorecard of the toxins you can be exposed to.

On awakening, you turn off the digital alarm clock by your bed and turn off your electric blanket. You turn on the television to see the morning news, and have a cup of coffee with a microwaved bagel. Perhaps you eat a bowl of cereal with milk topped with strawberries or a slice of toast. You may take vitamins or medications as part of your daily routine.

In the bathroom, you use the toilet, with a handy air freshener available, and take a shower or bath, washing with soap and shampoo. Then you apply body lotion, deodorant, and a scented body splash, cologne, or perfume. You brush your teeth with your electric toothbrush and gargle with mouthwash. You may wash with a separate facial cleanser and follow this up with a moisturizer, toner, and sun block. To style your artificially colored hair, you use your electric dryer and some hair spray for that final touch. You then dress in fresh clothes from the dry cleaner.

Women may put on makeup, including foundation, powder and blush, lip liner and lipstick, eye liner, shadow, and mascara; much of this will be reapplied many times a day. Men will usually shave with an electric shaver or use gels or foams prior to manual shaving, followed by the application of aftershave lotion.

You make a sandwich with lettuce and tomato for your lunch, cook breakfast for your children on your nonstick Teflon pan, and then leave for work by entering the garage through a convenient access door from the house. Outside, your lawn company is spraying weed killer on your perfectly manicured grass. You remember that, last week, the pest control company sprayed the interior of your house to get rid of termites. You get into your car where you automatically turn on the air conditioner or heater. Finally, you are off to work, hi ho, hi ho.

Here is the scorecard of potential toxins you just exposed yourself to in the above scenario.

In the bedroom and bathroom, you received artificial electromagnetic fields from your alarm clock, electric blanket, electric toothbrush, electric shaver, and electric hair dryer (as well as the microwave in your kitchen). Outgassing exposure came from the flame-retardant chemicals in your mattress (polybrominated diphenyl ethers); your synthetic carpet that was treated with benzene and styrene; your dry cleaned clothes that contained trichloroethylene and n-hexane (chemicals known to cause nerve cell damage, memory loss, and cardiac abnormalities); the chemicals from your furniture and wall paint; and all highly concentrated within your well-insulated bedroom and bathroom.

The insecticide that was sprayed to combat termites is also contained within this energy-efficient insulation. This ensures that you received a high degree exposure to the lethal chemical throughout the week after the spraying was done.

In your bathroom, the tap water in the sink and shower was laced with fluoride and chlorine in addition to traces of prescription drugs, steroids, antibiotics, and pesticides from your municipal water supply. The shower also liberated small amounts of chlorine and the other chemicals into the air, for you to inhale further and absorb into your body. The deodorizer under the toilet seat lid outgassed benzene fumes (capable of causing leukemia) while the air freshener plugged into the wall and your soap similarly dispersed phthalates (lowers sperm motility in adult men and is correlated with abdominal obesity and insulin resistance in men).

In the kitchen, the bowl of cereal and the toast you ate were made from genetically modified foods (discussed later in this chapter) and a dozen chemical food additives, including artificial sweeteners linked to a wide range of allergies and illnesses. The milk you poured into your bowl and the meat you placed in your sandwich contained synthetic hormones and antibiotics (injected into the animals to increase their size or production of milk).

The lettuce and sliced tomato in your sandwich and the strawberries in your cereal each contained the residues of half a dozen different pesticides. Wrapping it in plastic released vinyl chloride, a carcinogen known to cause liver, brain, and lung cancers. The Teflon pan was manufactured with Serum Perfluorooctanoic Acid (PFOA), which can cause hormone disruption (particularly thyroid dysfunction) and reproductive abnormalities in animal and human studies (this chemical is widely used in industrial and consumer products from stain- and water-resistant coatings for carpets and fabrics to fast-food packaging, fire-resistant foams, paints, and hydraulic fluids, according to the Organization for Economic Co-operation and Development).

When you left the house, opening the door to the garage created a vacuum effect, drawing inside all the fumes from the gasoline, paint cans, cleaning solvents, pesticides, and other chemicals located there. When a house is taller and warmer than the garage, this air is pulled inside and drawn upward just like a chimney, so the garage's plethora of contaminants becomes the house's breathing air. Outside, herbicides such as atrazine were spread all over the lawn your kids will play in after school.

The smell from your car, particularly when running the air conditioner on hot days, is from inhaling volatile organic compounds (VOCs), composed of cancer-causing chemicals such as styrene and formaldehyde.

Finally, add to your toxic scorecard are all the personal-care products you used. The Environmental Working Group estimates that every customer each day uses an average of nine personal-care products containing 126 separate ingredients, with at least one-third of these ingredients identified as causing cancer or other serious health problems.

Your mouthwash mixture included four active ingredients and half a dozen flavorings and coloring chemicals; the plastic bottle also leached its own chemicals into the mixture, which will be discussed below. The toothpaste contained fluoride, a known toxin (have you read the warning label lately on your tube of toothpaste?). Your deodorant contained seven chemicals including aluminum, parabens (a preservative), propylene glycol (a lubricant and suspected cancer agent), and other chemicals disguised under the term "fragrance." Your cologne or perfume also contained these "fragrance" chemicals, which are closely guarded secrets within the industry. The term "fragrance" covers chemicals that are linked to reproductive damage, hormone disruption, and can trigger allergic reactions. (Diethyl phthalate is one such chemical found in 97 percent of Americans and is linked to abnormal development of reproductive organs in baby boys and sperm damage in adult men. It is also linked to attention deficit disorder in children following mother's exposure prenatally).

Your skin lotions contained penetration-enhancing chemicals to drive the toxins deeper into your skin. If used, the cosmetics you placed on your face and in your nail polish have a 65 percent chance of containing carcinogenic ingredients (but only 11 percent have even been tested).

Widespread Toxicity

Like the Roman elite who unknowingly poisoned themselves with their lead cooking pots and utensils, modern-day man is being unknowingly contaminated by hundreds of products that provide a wealth of convenience, fun, and comfort. Modern progress has come at a deadly price: despite the most advanced technology in the world, our society's overall health has degenerated at an alarming and rapid pace.

We are awash in an ocean of industrial pollutants. There are 85,000 chemicals in commercial use in the United States, with 2000 added annually and the problem is that we really don't know most of the associated health effects. Even though these toxic substances are shown to accumulate in our fat, bones, blood, and organs, or pass through us in breast milk, urine, feces, sweat, semen, hair, and nails, the vast majority of chemicals have not been tested.

The Toxic Substances Control Act (TSCA) of 1976 allows chemicals to be sold and used unless they are proven to be a risk. It grandfathered many chemicals already in use without scrutiny, including Bisphenol A, bromated flame-retardants (polybrominated diphenyl ethers), and plastic softeners called phthalates (which, as mentioned in the toxic scorecard above, wreaks multiple kinds of havoc in men's bodies).

The United States, unlike the 27-member European Union (EU) does not operate under the "precautionary principle." The EU believes that, if the accumulation of evidence of a particular chemical (whether it is found in cosmetics, toys, appliances, or food) suggests a potential to cause harm, it will remove it from circulation in favor of preventing harm before it happens. It is one of the EU's main environmental and health policy regulatory tools and serves as a foundation for several international agreements.

But the Environmental Protection Agency (EPA) will not act until they have conclusive scientific evidence of toxic exposure, which is essentially the "prove harm" approach. The EPA must prove that a toxic substance "presents an unreasonable risk of injury to health or the environment" before they will regulate it.

The bar for this standard is set too high. It is extremely difficult to evaluate every chemical that is introduced each year for its toxic effect, not to mention the potential toxic interactions these chemicals may pose when combined with any of the other 85,000 chemicals. The EPA relies on research done by companies directly profiting from these chemicals to determine their safety. This is demonstrated in a 2005 report by the Government Accountability Office (the investigative arm of the U.S. Congress) that showed chemical companies provided health data to the EPA for only 15 percent of the thousands of new synthetic chemicals that have been introduced into the marketplace. Is the fox ever considered to be reliable when guarding the henhouse?

This is similar to the open-door policy of the Food and Drug Administration (FDA) when it comes to cosmetics and personal-care products. Under FDA regulations, with the exception of a pre-marketing review for color additives, neither cosmetic products nor the ingredients used are reviewed or approved by the FDA before being sold to the public. The FDA has estimated that 65 percent of women's cosmetics contain potentially carcinogenic ingredients, yet 87 percent of the ingredients in personal-care products have not been assessed for safety by the Cosmetic Ingredient Review, the industry's self-policing safety panel. According to the Environmental Working Group, an analysis of ingredients found more than half of cosmetic products contained estrogen-like chemicals that can disrupt hormones in the body.

Also, the use of the word "fragrance" in personal-care products denotes a pleasing smell from a seemingly innocuous green environment but behind this pleasant façade lurks a chemical sinkhole. Companies are able to keep the chemicals that constitute "fragrance" as a trade secret because the *Federal Fair Packaging and Labeling Act* of 1973, which requires cosmetic ingredients to be listed on product labels, explicitly exempts fragrances (even though the fragrance industry has 3100 stock chemical ingredients). As a result, people using perfume, cologne, body spray, and other scented cosmetics like lotion and aftershave are unknowingly exposed to "scent" chemicals as well as chemicals found in the products' solvents, stabilizers, UV absorbers (used to increase to stability and shelf life), preservatives, and dyes that may increase their risk of health problems.

Chemicals found in the products may increase their risk of health problems.

For example, a recent study commissioned by the Campaign for Safe Cosmetics, and analyzed by Environmental Working Group, revealed 38 secret chemicals in 17 name brand fragrance products with an average of 14 secret chemicals per product (see Table 8.1). An average of 10 chemicals per product were known sensitizers that trigger allergic reactions (fragrance is now considered among the top five allergens in North America and European countries; see Table 8.2). In fact, in 2007, the American Contact Dermatitis Society named fragrance "Allergen of the Year."

In addition, four "hormone disruptor" chemicals were found per product. These chemicals act as hormone disruptors by interfering with the production, release, transport, metabolism, and binding of hormones to their targets in the body (see table 8.3). They have been linked to a wide range of health problems including an increased risk of breast and prostate cancers, reproductive toxicity and effects on the developing fetus, and predisposition to metabolic disease such as thyroid problems.

Similarly, there are many other daily household products that contain strongly scented, volatile ingredients hidden behind the word "fragrance" with increased health risks. These include shampoos, lotions, bath products, cleaning sprays, air fresheners, candles, toys, and laundry and dishwashing detergents. Many of these products bear claims like "natural fragrance," "pure fragrance," or "organic fragrance." The problem is that none of these terms have an enforceable legal definition and are misleading. In fact, one study found that 82 percent of perfumes based on "natural ingredients" contained synthetic fragrances. Even an "unscented" or "fragrance-free" personal-care product may contain a "masking fragrance," a mixture of chemicals meant to cover the odor of other ingredients.

The United States is far behind other industrialized countries when it comes to cosmetic safety. To date, the FDA has banned or restricted 11 chemicals for use in cosmetics, in contrast to 1100 chemicals banned or restricted from cosmetics sold in the EU. You can find a list of 200 companies that have fully disclosed all ingredients, including fragrance, on their ingredient labels. These ingredients are also listed in EWG's Skin Deep Cosmetics Database as part of their commitment to the Compact for Safe Cosmetics, a pledge of safety and transparency administered by the Campaign for Safe Cosmetics. Learn more at http://safecosmetics.org/compact.

The FDA is also responsible for oversight of new drugs and food additives, but in making decisions it relies upon the drug and food manufacturers for safety information.

The net result from these policies is that many substances banned in Europe are still in widespread use in the United States, leading to a reverse double standard. Having inverted the goals of our forefathers to provide for the protection of our citizens, we are now being left behind in the toxic dust, literally, by the rest of the world.

In 1987, the EPA estimated that each of us carry, on average, 700 toxins in our body! It is a womb-to-grave exposure; contamination begins at conception through the mother's body burden (the total amount of a chemical or its metabolites) that she already carries. A 2004 study by the Environmental Working Group found, in ten randomly chosen babies born in the United States, the umbilical-cord blood contained 287 chemicals worthy of a chemical dump site. Of these, 180 were known to cause cancer, 217 were neurotoxins, and 208 caused birth defects in animal tests.

Add up all the synthetic chemicals laced throughout our meals including genetically modified, processed, and fast food, toxins from medicines, personal-care products, cosmetics, consumer electronics, household furniture, and building supplies, and this pre-existing contamination in the womb. You may begin to appreciate how we acquired the total body burden each of us carries through the common and minute exposures that we experience in our daily lives.

Although the father of toxicology, Paracelsus, coined the axiom "the dose makes the poison" in the sixteenth century to denote how a higher dose produces a greater effect, this does not hold true with today's toxic chemicals. Many synthetic chemicals are biologically active at incredibly low levels. As well, the synergy (the simultaneous action of two or more chemicals in which the total effect is much greater than the sum of their individual effects) between two or more chemicals will produce additional toxic effects. This can occur even when the individual contaminants, when measured, have a toxicity deemed too low to pose a health threat.

The alarm bell about the impact of these synergies was first raised by Rachel Carson in her 1962 book *Silent Spring* about the toxic effects on health of "two or more different carcinogens acting together." She revealed that the powerful pesticide DDT was not just killing insects and irrevocably harming birds and wildlife but also boomerangs back to us through contamination of the entire world food supply.

The Centers for Disease Control (CDC) has been monitoring our body burden in the largest ongoing study of chemical exposures ever conducted on humans. In 2008, the CDC evaluated the presence of 212 chemicals in the blood and urine of 2400 participants in its National Health and Nutrition

Examination Survey (NHANES). As reported in the *Fourth National Report on Human Exposure to Environmental Chemicals,* dozens of toxins were found in every single test subject.

However, these results do not come close to measuring the participants' real body burden. For every chemical and pesticide measured, there are hundreds more for which there is no current method to screen for their presence in human tissues. That's how rampant and how pervasive these toxins are. The plastics we use, the water we drink, the food we eat, the showers we take, the toiletries and cosmetics we use, and the products we clean our homes with are loaded with harmful chemicals.

None of the above takes into account the additional toxic burden from the contaminated air we breathe, inside and outside our homes.

Toxins are one of your biggest physical stressors. They wreak havoc with your hormones, initiating the stress response that elevates your cortisol levels and creates free radicals that damage your cells and DNA. Simply put, if your body is loaded with toxins this will prematurely age you and lead to autoimmunity, neurodegenerative diseases, cancers, diabetes…you name it, the list expands with each passing decade.

A 2005 National Institute of Health report, *Progress in Autoimmune Diseases Research,* pronounced that 23.5 million people (1 in 12 Americans, 80 percent of whom are women) are now afflicted by one or more of the nearly 100 known autoimmune diseases, and 40 million people will soon fall ill because it takes several years for an autoimmune disorder to develop. This is the second-leading cause of chronic disease, leading to an average 15-year reduction in an afflicted person's life.

It is estimated that a quarter of the American population carries a genetic susceptibility to autoimmunity that may one day be triggered by exposure to one toxin too many, resulting in a total-body toxin overload. Donna Jackson Nakazawa, author of *The Autoimmune Epidemic,* describes the threshold at which autoimmune disease finally develops as "the barrel effect." A barrel, filled with water at the rim, doesn't spill until one small drop of liquid is added; then the water cascades over the sides. In the same way, a person's genetic "barrel" or body burden gets filled up with susceptible genes, hormones, environmental toxins, and infections until just one more hit, such as a virus or other environmental trigger, causes a cascading effect of immune system overload. It ultimately manifests as an autoimmune disorder such as rheumatoid arthritis, multiple sclerosis, lupus, asthma, or thousands of subclinical symptoms that fall into the general category of environmental allergies.

Environmental toxins are highly absorbable through your skin and many will bioaccumulate throughout your lifetime. Even low levels of exposure will disrupt your hormone systems, decrease fertility, and weaken your immune systems. That's why most anti-aging doctors I know will not put any pesticides or herbicides on their lawn.

But consider that, when you swim in a chlorinated pool or take a shower with unfiltered water, you are absorbing a lot of that chlorine through your skin. In a ten-minute shower, the toxin absorption can be equivalent to drinking eight glasses of chlorinated water; and chlorine is linked to bladder and rectal cancer. In addition, depending on your diet, you can absorb toxins through your food. These will accumulate in your stomach and intestines and migrate through your blood into all of your organs. And like a West Virginia coal miner, you also absorb toxins by inhaling them. They come from exhaust fumes, airborne industrial particulates, and chemicals being off-gassed in various ways within your home.

Many native religions, it is believed that man cannot be separated from nature as we are all part of the same grand ecosystem.

In many native religions, it is believed that man cannot be separated from nature as we are all part of the same grand ecosystem. According to such beliefs, the environment is not only outside us but within us. It seems they are correct because the same poisons running through our rivers, lakes, and oceans are also running through our bodies. There is no safe island in the world where one may go to avoid these toxins; it has become a global problem.

Toxin exposure took center stage following the 2008-2009 Annual Report submission of President Obama's Cancer Panel (a body of experts reporting directly to President Obama). This report stated that widespread exposure to environmental carcinogens was causing "grievous harm" to Americans, which the country's National Cancer Program had not addressed. According to this report, the 34,000 cancer deaths estimated by the American Cancer Society to be caused by environmental pollutants were "grossly underestimated" due to lack of research.

The report urged the Obama administration to act by using the power of his office to remove the carcinogens and other toxins from food, water, and air, even if the evidence linking cancer to these chemicals wasn't definitive. It recommended "the adoption of the precautionary principle as the cornerstone of a new cancer prevention strategy that emphasizes primary prevention, redirects accordingly both research and policy agendas, and sets tangible goals for reducing or eliminating toxic environmental exposures implicated in cancer causation."

We may be turning the corner on the unregulated use of industrial chemicals with the proposed *Safe Chemicals Act* (formally the *Kid-Safe Chemicals Act*) introduced in the 110th U.S. Congress. It is a good first step in reforming the laws and forcing companies to prove that their chemicals are child-safe before they are put on the market. The establishment of new research programs will help us to better understand the risk that toxic industrial chemicals pose to children.

M a l e v o l e n t   M e t a l s

Heavy metals disrupt your cell metabolism. They slowly collect in your body, irritate your cells, and can literally wipe out your immune system. For example, ingesting mercury activates an autoimmune response, leading to various autoimmune disorders. Heavy-metal toxicity is a health disaster of epidemic proportions in our society.

Arsenic, lead, mercury, and other toxic rubble are all found in our food supply. For example, chicken feed is known to contain arsenic, lead, and other heavy metals. So you and the chickens ingest these poisonous substances. Organic, free-range chickens are raised without the use of contaminated feed.

Every fish in the world is now contaminated with mercury. The bigger the fish, the greater the contamination: kingfish, swordfish, tuna, and mackerel are all unsafe to eat. Probably the least contaminated large fish is wild salmon from the Aleutian Islands, but even its flesh contains a small amount of mercury.

With long-term exposure, eventually your brain will not work right and you end up with dementia. Pregnant women are told not to eat any fish because mercury can concentrate in the fetus' brain and retard its mental or physical development. In fact, 60,000 children are born brain injured from fish-related mercury exposure every year. Mercury also oxidizes LDL cholesterol, leading to the beginning stages of coronary artery disease.

However, fish oil is a great source of omega-3 fatty acid, which helps to balance your hormones and reduce inflammation, among other benefits. To counteract the effect of mercury contamination, choose a high-level, "micronized" fish oil supplement because cheaper, mass-produced brands are loaded with mercury. Flax seed oil, primrose oil, nuts, berries, and whole grains are other sources of omega-3 fatty acids.

Organic beef has a higher concentration of nutrients with roughly a sixth the amount of pesticides.

Cows ingest petrochemicals, pesticides, herbicides, mercury, PCBs, and other chemicals from their feed, which then bioaccumulates. They are injected with growth hormones and antibiotics to make them fat for the marketplace. Consuming this beef adds to the toxic load in your body. In contrast, organic beef has a higher concentration of nutrients with roughly a sixth the amount of pesticides.

Organic produce has a similarly low level of toxins. But with inorganic produce, as discussed in chapter 4, the Environmental Working Group's analysis of data collected from the US Department of Agriculture between 2000 and 2007 clearly depicts the toxic residue.

Eat organic foods as much as you can. Toxins don't just go away; they become concentrated in your body. Fortunately, since your body is 75 percent water, you can excrete soluble toxins by following a healthy diet and good hydration.

But most of these toxins are fat soluble, which means that they either cannot be excreted or it is achieved with great difficulty and at the cost of depleting many other essential nutrients.

Eating contaminated food leads to loss of integrity in the intestinal wall lining and "leaky gut syndrome." Increased permeability of the intestinal wall allows small food particles and bacteria to enter the blood system. The immune system creates antibodies against them, so that large numbers of different foods now set off an immune reaction when they are eaten. These antibodies may also attack any cells that are structurally similar to food molecules, leading to autoimmune diseases. Other ramifications include poor absorption of nutrients, impaired immunity in the gut, and "translocation" of gut bacteria via the bloodstream into other parts of the body.

Genetically modified (GM) foods involve genetic engineering; genes from a completely different species are inserted into the DNA of a plant (or animal). These genetically modified organisms (GMO), which I like to call Frankenstein foods, are exceptionally bad news. The organism's entire DNA is altered and disrupted along with the environment in which it is expressed. But the FDA's assessment of GM foods has been based on the idea of "substantial equivalence." In a 1992 report, it stated "if a new food is found to be substantially equivalent in composition and nutritional characteristics to an existing food, it can be regarded as safe as the conventional food."

The FDA's stance is that GM foods are substantially equivalent to unmodified, "natural" foods, and therefore not subject to FDA regulation. However, as we've learned from the international Human Genome Project (2003), there are only 23,688 genes in the body but they are "expressed" in three million different ways through single nucleotide polymorphisms (SNPs). The expression depends on what you feel, eat, and experience in your environment, and within this scenario GMOs can lead to unpredictable results.

Forcing a foreign gene into an organism may cause other native genes to stop expressing certain proteins or enzymes (known as "gene silencing") and/or increase the expression of others, causing an imbalance. Some genes may express themselves in unanticipated ways, such as allergens or toxins. Not enough research has been done to fully realize the implications, even though

GM crops were widely introduced in 1996, and more than 60 percent of the processed foods on supermarket shelves contain derivatives of the eight available GM foods: soy, corn oil from canola and cottonseed, sugar from sugar beets, Hawaiian papaya, and a small amount of zucchini, alfalfa, and crookneck squash (yet another reason to eat organic, whole foods).

In addition, more than 80 percent of mass-market cheese is made with chymosin produced by genetically modified microorganisms. Most of the meat, poultry, and eggs sold in supermarkets come from animals fed genetically modified feed.

According to The American Academy of Environmental Medicine (AAEM), animal studies reveal that GMOs cause a long list of disorders including "infertility, immune dysregulation, accelerated aging, dysregulation of genes associated with cholesterol synthesis, faulty insulin regulation, cell signaling, and protein formation, and changes in the liver, kidney, spleen and gastrointestinal system." In May 2009, the AAEM called on the U.S. government to implement an immediate moratorium on all GM foods and urged physicians to prescribe non-GMO diets for their patients. Their concerns included the mounting, negative experimental data from animal testing.

The AAEM believed that it was imperative to adopt the European precautionary principle to regulate the use of GM foods. The data showed that GM foods pose a serious health risk in the areas of toxicology, allergy, and immune function, and reproductive, metabolic, physiological, and genetic health. Even world-renowned biologist Dr. Pushpa M. Bhargava, after reviewing 600 scientific journals, concluded that GMOs are a major contributor to the sharply deteriorating health of Americans.

Genetically modified foods are known to cause allergic reactions such as eczema, asthma, and respiratory ailments. It happened in England when GM soy was introduced: soy allergies skyrocketed by 50 percent. The process of creating a GMO can introduce new allergens, elevate existing ones, and provoke sensitivities to previously harmless non-GM foods.

Our bodies have 10 trillion cells but there are 100 trillion bacteria in our gut, which makes up 70 percent of our immune system. In the only published human study about a GM food (soy) to date, it revealed that foreign genes from these "frankenfoods" were being incorporated into the DNA of the human gut bacteria. A GM meal was fed to seven subjects who wore a colostomy bag because part of their lower bowel had been removed in a previous operation. Scientists took bacteria from the stools in the colostomy bag and cultivated them. In three of the seven samples, they found bacteria had taken up an herbicide-resistant gene from the GM food.

This horizontal transfer of DNA from GM plants to bacteria in the gut has disturbing implications. It could result in new viruses and bacteria that cause diseases, spread drug and antibiotic resistance among pathogens, or trigger cancer by jumping into genomes of mammalian cells. For corn crops inserted with genes from the soil bacterium *Bacillus Thuringiensis,* which produces an insect-killing pesticide Cry1Ab protein (commonly called Bt-toxin) in every cell of the plant, these genes could transform our own gut flora into living pesticide factories for the duration of our lives.

We don't know what the full implications may be. However, because they have "substantially equivalent" status, these genetically engineered products are not required by food regulations in the United States to be segregated or labeled. (GM foods are required to be labeled in Europe, Australia, and Japan). As we have seen in other industries, the FDA does not oversee and approve GM foods before they are allowed on the market. The FDA puts the responsibility on the food companies developing the GM food to indicate that they are safe for human consumption. Unfortunately, we are now the experimental canaries in the coal mine and it could be many generations in the future before we realize how we've contaminated and poisoned ourselves and our offspring with these "frankenfoods."

Since GM ingredients in packaged or canned foods are not labeled in the U.S, there is no way of knowing if the food you buy has been genetically modified. In addition, if grain is not labeled GM, how can you be certain that you are eating organic eggs, dairy, and meat? Even with packaged foods that have nutritional labeling, the accuracy is suspect. The FDA saddled manufacturers with the responsibility for assuring the validity of nutritional information in their products. But according to government guidelines, the nutrition label has to be off by more than 20 percent before it violates federal law!

It is the FDA's responsibility to oversee the accuracy of nutrition labeling for up to 80 percent of packaged foods in the United States. But the Government Accountability Office (GAO) gave the FDA a failing grade for not preventing false and inaccurate product labeling in an October 2008 report, stating that the FDA hasn't kept up with enforcement efforts. Although the number of food products has increased dramatically in the last few years, random sampling of nutrition labels has not been performed by the FDA since the 1990s; and the FDA does not track the correction of known violations.

To ensure that you age well, buy organic foods and ingredients and prepare home-cooked meals. Organically grown foods cannot be genetically modified (but they may be contaminated by GM food grown nearby) and you can control the ingredients. You can distinguish between fruits and vegetables that are commercially grown, genetically modified, or organically grown by the stickers on the produce. If there is no sticker, look at the sign for a four- or five-digit number. If the number has four digits, it's conventionally grown. If it has five digits and begins with an 8, it's genetically modified. If it has five digits and begins with a 9, it's organically grown.

Airborne Disease

One of my law school professors died of dioxin poison emitted by the trash-burning power plant near his home. It was located about two miles away. No one in Columbus, Ohio realized how it could poison their systems; everyone thought that burning trash would help reduce the load on our landfill. The problem with burning trash is that we breathe in the same air. Too late it was discovered that dioxin, which the EPA says is "known to be a carcinogen to humans," was poisoning the community's air.

The Dioxin Homepage (ejnet.org/dioxin) states that dioxin was the primary toxic component in manufacturing the military's cancer-causing Agent Orange; it was found at Love Canal in Niagara Falls, NY; and it was the basis for evacuations at Times Beach, MO and in Seveso, Italy. Major sources of dioxin in our environment are waste-burning incinerators, backyard trash burning, tree burning, and byproducts in exhaust fumes from diesel trucks and buses. Other sources include industrial manufacturing of bleached fibers in paper and textiles, the production of wood preservatives, chlorinated pesticides and herbicides, and the manufacturing process of virtually every type of plastic and bleached or resin-coated food packaging found in supermarkets.

There is no known safe level of exposure to this virulent chemical. I personally believe that this airborne carcinogen led to the esophageal cancer that killed my former professor at the age of 43.

Another source of air contamination is coal-burning power plants. Reported at msnbc.msn.com, a 2004 study linked coal-plant emissions to lung cancer, asthma, and heart attacks. The EPA reports that coal-burning power plants comprise the largest human-sourced mercury emissions into the air in the U.S., which amounts to about 50 tons of mercury each year. This represents 33 percent of total U.S. emissions, with municipal and medical waste incinerators contributing 19 percent and 10 percent, respectively. About 25 percent of these emissions are deposited within the country; the rest enters the global climate cycle.

Human-made sources account for 60 percent of worldwide air emissions, with volcanic eruptions and emissions from the oceans accounting for the other 40 percent. These dry particles of mercury travel thousands of miles from their source of origin, across the American landscape, leaving deposits in lakes, rivers, parks, forests, and communities. They contaminate fish, birds, mammals, and people.

They settle onto your front porch. You breathe these toxins in, which lodge in your lungs and never leave. You step in the residue, and track it onto your living room rug. Then your baby crawls in it, and he absorbs the toxins.

The atmosphere is implicated in many contaminations. Lead, arsenic, and other heavy metals may be carried by wind from contaminated sediment in wind-blown dust from lakes and rivers, diesel fuel (which emits one-third of all nitrogen oxide and a quarter of all particulate matter emissions from mobile sources), and wood smoke.

Perfluorinated chemicals (PFCs), an ingredient in the fluoropolymers found in microwave popcorn bags, stain-free carpets, fast-food wrappers, denture cleaners, and windshield-wiper fluid (within five years of introduction), have been found everywhere in the world, including the blood of polar bears and seals in the Arctic, thousands of miles from any possible industrial source. How could this chemical become so ubiquitous so soon? Researchers believe the atmosphere is the cause.

Molecules of toxic chemicals attach themselves to dust particles and travel the upper air currents north to colder climates, which draw them in like a magnet. Marla Cone, in her 2005 book *Silent Snow: The Slow Poisoning of the Arctic,* identifies at least 200 synthetic chemicals that are adversely affecting the health of indigenous people at the top of the world.

Indoors and outdoors, airborne pollution is actively bringing disease causing chemicals to snuggle deeply into your tissues. Your new car smell comes from the the toxins off-gassing from the plastics inside the car. The new rug you installed in your home is off-gassing loads of petrochemical toxins that you will then absorb into your lungs.

Carpeting can cause additional problems from being exposed over time to humidity and moisture, human and animal dander, and dirt. This does not include what happens during the aging process as the toxic particulate matter from which the carpeting is made breaks down and becomes distributed into your breathing air.

The home has about 250 times the amount of toxins as exist outdoors. One major problem is insulation: it keeps the cold out, and all the toxins stay in. This includes chemicals from deodorants and hair sprays, off-gassing from furniture and construction materials, carbon monoxide, pet dander, radon, and mold, all of which accumulates inside. One way to reduce this toxic accumulation is to open the windows and air out your home, even during the winter months.

Radon and carbon monoxide detectors are essential in helping you avoid exposure to indoor toxins. In addition, ensure that your garage is well ventilated because many chemicals tend to be stored there. Each time you open your door, and particularly when you have a door from the garage to the inside of your home, they all come pouring inside.

Also, use a good air purifier to capture airborne particles. Houseplants are a natural filter; they are said to remove about 87 percent of particulates and toxins. One houseplant can clean about 100 square feet of air, so have plants in every room.

The toxins and the chemicals from dry cleaning your clothes will sit inside that plastic bag until you put them in your closet and expose yourself to the toxic trichloroethylene used to clean them. These days, I air out any dry-cleaned clothes in my garage or outdoors before bringing them into my home.

Water   Works

The worst toxins found in both tap and certain bottled waters are byproducts created during the disinfection process. Trihalomethanes (TMMs) and haloacetic acids (HAAS) are formed when chlorine reacts with natural organic matter such as decaying vegetation in the source water during water treatment. They are about 10,000 times more toxic than the chlorine that creates them. Use an activated carbon filter to remove them from your drinking water.

Trihalomethanes are classified as "group-B carcinogens," which means that they're known to cause cancer in laboratory animals. They are linked to reproductive problems in animals and humans, and one study suggests that lifetime consumption of chlorine-treated water more than doubles the risk of bladder and rectal cancers in some individuals. Limited studies of haloacetic acids suggest similar risks.

When talking specifically about bottled water, surveys indicate that 35 percent of consumers believe that bottled water is safer than tap water. Nothing could be further from the truth. It is estimated that 40 percent of bottled water is just regular tap water. This makes bottled water a very expensive proposition, given the fact that we are paying 1900 times more for it compared to drinking water out of our household tap.

In one test performed by the Environmental Working Group, 38 low-level contaminants were found in bottled water, with each of the 10 tested brands containing an average of eight chemicals. More than one-third of the chemicals found are not regulated in bottled water. They include disinfection byproducts, caffeine, acetaminophen, heavy metals, and minerals including arsenic and radioactive isotopes; fertilizer residue (nitrate and ammonia); and a broad range of other, tentatively identified industrial chemicals used as solvents, plasticizers, viscosity decreasing agents, and propellants. In contrast, testing by water utilities has found 315 pollutants in the tap water Americans drink, according to the Environmental Working Group.

In addition, the consumption of these bottled waters is polluting our world. Increasing amounts of these non-biodegradable plastic water bottles end up in our landfills and in our waters. There is a great Pacific garbage patch that is described as the eighth continent because it contains 100 million tons of trash, bags, toys, and plastic bottles in an area twice the size of the United States. It is the planet's largest garbage dump measuring about 10 million square miles down to a depth of 30 meters. It is held together by a whirling vortex of current that has collected so much debris in the last 50 years, it has been measured to have six pounds of plastic for every pound of plankton. A United Nations 2006 office estimated that every square mile of ocean contains on average 46,000 pieces of floating plastic. It litters the beaches and rivers, washing up on Hawaii and other islands, although the majority of it stays in the water, poisoning marine life and the poisons ultimately end up on our dinner plate.

According to a U.S. Conference of Mayors' resolution passed in 2007, water bottle production in the U.S. uses 1.5 million barrels of oil per year, which is enough energy to power 250,000 homes or fuel 100,000 cars for a year. Approximately 2.5 million tons of carbon dioxide is produced in the manufacturing of plastic bottles per year.

Chemicals leaching from these bottles into the water include bisphenol-A (BPA), a toxin found in hard, clear plastic used to make everything from baby bottles and dental sealants to epoxy resins and food packaging. BPAs have been shown to cause genetic abnormalities in mice and humans; it may be linked to long-term fertility problems, earlier sexual development in females, decreased sperm count in males, and increases in neurodevelopment disorders such as attention deficit hyperactivity disorder, autism, breast and prostate cancers, and childhood obesity.

A recent study found that exposure to high levels of BPA may increase the risk of erectile dysfunction and other sexual problems in men. The study, reported by CNN.com on November 11, 2009, compared the rates of sexual dysfunction in two groups of workers in China: 230 men who were exposed to BPA, at levels about 50 times higher than average, through their work in factories, and some 400 men, including workers in other industries, who were not exposed to abnormally high levels of BPA. Men exposed to the BPA were four times as likely to suffer from erectile dysfunction and seven times as likely to have difficulty ejaculating.

BPA's use is so widespread that the U.S. Center for Disease Control and Prevention found BPA in the urine of 93 percent of the people tested. Use of this chemical is out of control: more than six billion pounds of BPAs per year are used by industry, primarily in the production of polycarbonate plastics and toxic resins used to coat metal products such as food cans, bottle tops, and water supply pipes.

Heat helps to release toxic chemicals from the plastic bottle directly into the water it's supposed to keep pure. The bottles are subjected to extreme temperatures during warehouse storage and truck transportation; temperatures can reach 150 degrees Fahrenheit. This all happens before you, the consumer, can buy and drink the toxic contents. Then, if you leave bottled water in your car on a hot summer day, you help to release these chemicals.

A better suggestion is to install a reverse osmosis filtering system in your home, or use inexpensive activated charcoal filters, and drink this water from steel bottles.

Environmental Toxins

Environmental estrogens are chemical compounds including the pesticide DDT, BPA, and dioxane (used in grooming products). These are estrogen mimics, or xenoestrogens, which are chemicals that act like estrogens in the body. We ingest them due to various types of environmental contamination. There are environmental estrogens in our cosmetics and grooming products and throughout our food supply, including the plastic containers used to package foods.

These artificial and synthetic estrogens disrupt the body's hormonal balance, leading to a wide range of physiological disorders and diseases. Personal-care products are chock full of them: 57 percent of all products contain paraben preservatives, nearly 2 percent contain surfactants called alkylphenols, and just over 2 percent contain estrogenic sunscreen ingredients, according to a 2004 product assessment by the Environmental Working Group.

For women, such chemicals are linked to early onset of puberty and increased risk for endometrial and breast cancer, Type II diabetes, cardiovascular disease, and polycystic ovarian syndrome. There is plenty of evidence that environmental estrogens are also harming men, including decreased sperm count, sexual dysfunctions, and prostate and testicular cancer.

Other harmful effects include increases in neurodevelopment disorders, such as attention deficit hyperactivity disorder and autism, and childhood obesity. These chemicals are seriously harming our children.

There is ample evidence that boys and girls are both entering puberty at increasingly younger ages, some girls as early as the age of seven (the full journey to sexual maturity takes an average of two years). This alarming shortening of their childhood is linked in part to environmental toxins. Early puberty has been shown to raise the risk of breast cancer and polycystic ovary syndrome in women, low sperm counts and sexual dysfunction in men, and emotional disorders including high-risk and addictive behaviors in later adolescence.

The Breast Cancer Fund, a publicly funded advocacy group, commissioned *The Falling Age of Puberty*, a comprehensive review of existing research. Published in 2007 by ecologist Sandra Steingraber, it describes early-onset puberty as an ecological disorder caused by various environmental influences including exposure to pollutants, plastics, and chemicals.

For women, early-onset puberty means they will end up hitting menopause earlier. This poses some increased risks of cancer. A woman's body contains a finite number of eggs, and the sooner they're gone, the earlier into menopause she will go.

Environmental toxins also affect your thyroid hormones. The thyroid contains the highest concentration of iodine in the body. Toxins displace the iodine, interfering with production of its two main hormones. This makes the thyroid very sluggish, leading to a hypothyroid condition.

If you brush your teeth with fluoride toothpaste, or eat mass-produced bread containing bromine, or ingest any of a hundred known toxins, your thyroid will be under stress. It takes an average of seven years before someone is diagnosed with hypothyroidism, during which time serious, irreversible damage can be done.

The pituitary gland is also extremely sensitive to toxins. It produces four major hormones and four stimulating hormones that signal the glands to release other hormones that regulate systems throughout your body. Environmental toxins cause the pituitary to become sluggish in manufacturing them.

The pineal gland, located in an area between your eyes, is also sensitive to toxins. It produces melatonin, which supports your adrenal glands. Melatonin is also the most potent antioxidant available. With low levels of melatonin, you don't receive this antioxidant benefit and you can't sleep well, which stresses your body.

The stress response exhausts your adrenal glands; increased, chronic inflammation causes more aches and pains; your thinking becomes impaired; concentration and focus decline; you gain weight; and semen count declines in men.

In effect, environmental toxicity has a global effect on your body. Trying to deal with the stress of toxic contamination can eventually lead to the breakdown of your entire immune system. You can end up with a hyperactive immune system that begins as a normal activation of the immune system but ends in an immune system network gone haywire.

Body-Enhancing Bioidenticals

Along with a special diet, certain neutriceuticals, and active cleansing of toxins, bioidentical hormones play their part in reversing autoimmunity. They support the immune system, which is one of the biggest benefits, helping you to fight the toxins that are attacking you.

Bioidentical hormones help to stabilize your body by filling your cells' receptors with a natural hormone, not with toxins from environmental contamination or synthetics found in most hormone medications. They are not nearly as concentrated as artificial hormones, and that's the reason they work so well. They gently restore balance throughout your body.

It's one reason why synthetic estrogen in the form of Premarin poses such a high risk for breast cancer, heart attacks, and strokes when bioidentical estrogen does not. Bioidentical hormones allow your body to work the way it should: reducing the stress effect from environmental and pharmaceutical toxins, lowering your cortisol levels, and inhibiting production of free radicals, all of which cause premature aging.

Because they are biologically identical to your hormones, they support the body's functions to restore your mental concentration and focus, deep cellular energy, libido and virility, refreshing sleep, and stable weight and soul-level well-being. A body that is more hormonally balanced simply functions better. It's more efficient in every way, and this including releasing toxins.

It improves your tolerance for the toxins we're all exposed to, and helps to eliminate them as much as possible. Bioidenticals are a body-enhancing way to deal with your toxic load. They are the body's immune enhancer, allowing it to function the way nature meant it to.

Bioidentical hormones also help you to shed excess weight, which is critical for mature health and hormonal balance. Fat cells aromatize testosterone into estrogen, causing hormonal imbalance, and fat is a storehouse of toxins. It is thought by many that obesity is the body's mechanism for safely compartmentalizing fat-soluble toxins.

You release fat-soluble toxins as you eliminate fat. But this is one reason why it's not advisable to lose more than one to two pounds a week. With a faster rate of weight loss, the toxic load being released becomes too high. You will absorb many of these toxins or experience other reactions such as dizziness, heart palpitations, headache, diarrhea, aches and pains, low joint pain, and so on. Good nutrition and drinking a lot of filtered water also helps the body to deal with toxins being released through weight loss.

Life-Saving Practices

Because our environment is so extensively polluted, I don't think we can ever get to zero in terms of toxic load. So you must keep your immune system functioning at its highest level and not let it be compromised. This includes reducing inflammation wherever possible.

An imbalance in your hormones becomes a source of inflammation in the body, which releases a lot of damaging, disease-causing free radicals. Another source is gastrointestinal disorders, such as leaky-gut and irritable-bowel syndromes. In addition to interfering with the absorption of nutrients, a healthy, strong digestion and elimination system are important for dealing with toxins.

Chelation is very effective for heavy-metal detoxification. It is the most effective method to remove these poisonous ores because they are stored in fat and it's difficult to get them released. I've seen children receive 30 to 40 chelation treatments and nothing appears to be working until the last three or so; then suddenly the lead, mercury, or other heavy metals start shooting out of the body. It then takes about 48 hours for the body to excrete these substances through the urine. This safe, medically supervised procedure, which has been in use for 40 years in the United States, delivers the chelate either orally or intravenously.

Chelation removes heavy metals from the bloodstream by means of a chelate such as ethylenediamine tetraacetic acid (EDTA), which attaches to metal molecules and escorts them out of the body through urine, stool, and sweat. EDTA is responsible for the reduction of intracellular heavy metals that impair enzyme reactions and block metabolic pathways. Heavy metal accumulation has been associated with Alzheimer's disease, Parkinson's disease, and cardiac arrhythmias.

Chelation decreases the risk for heart attacks and strokes by decreasing lead, which has been implicated as a silent killer in these chronic diseases. It is used intravenously to remove such metals as aluminum, cadmium, lead, and tin but is not very effective for removal of mercury or arsenic.

DiSodium EDTA (NaEDTA) is approved by the FDA for use in hypercalcemia and ventricular arrhythmias associated with digitalis toxicity. Calcium DiSodium EDTA (CaEDTA) is approved by the FDA for use in the removal of lead and other heavy metals. DMPS (2,3-dimercaptopropane-l-sylfonate) is another chelate that can be taken orally, intravenously, or in a suppository. It is used for removal of mercury, lead, arsenic, cadmium, nickel, tin, and other metals. DMSA (2,3,-dimercaptosuccinic acid) is another chelate that is usually given to remove mercury, lead, and arsenic from the body. It has a unique property not found in DMPS, which is the ability to chelate heavy metals from the brain. It can be given orally or rectally.

Chelation therapy has also been used off label for a variety of different diseases. These include coronary artery disease, Type I and Type II diabetes, arthrosclerosis, cerebral vascular disease, osteoarthritis, peripheral vascular disease, venous stasis disorders, cardiac arrhythmias, peripheral neuropathy, collagen vascular disease, fibromyalgia, Alzheimer's disease, osteoporosis, and Parkinson's disease.

You should be drinking, on a daily basis, half your weight in ounces to be property hydrated.

There are also herbal and nutritional chelators that can be used. Herbal chelators, which are effective at eliminating toxins, include burdock root, dandelion root, lemon balm, milk thistle, and uva ursi. Nutritional chelators also can be used as part of a biodetoxification program. These include glutathione, alpha lipoic acid, N-acetylcysteine (a precursor to glutathione), and cysteine.

Of course, lifestyle modification is required as part of a complete therapeutic program. This would include stress reduction, caffeine avoidance, alcohol limitation, smoking cessation, exercise, and nutritional counseling.

Fortunately, you can eliminate a lot of water-soluble toxins by drinking enough water. Good hydration allows your cells to flush out toxins and your body to excrete them. But it's been estimated that 70 percent of people are dehydrated because they don't drink enough water. I'm not talking about beverages loaded with high-fructose corn syrup, either: I'm talking about plain filtered water.

You should be drinking, on a daily basis, half your weight in ounces to be property hydrated. This means drink a quart of water for every 50 pounds you weigh every day, which is a lot of water.

Many people are chronically dehydrated. Instead of water, we're drinking carbonated and caffeinated drinks, which are highly concentrated in chemicals and sugars. These leach minerals from your cells and are also dehydrating. Intracellular dehydration leads to lower efficiency of the mitochondria, the energy makers in each cell. This leads to further toxin buildup and ultimately the death of these organelles.

When I see someone in the ER, especially an elderly person, who is very fatigued and weak with low energy, the first thing I do is load them with a liter of intravenous fluid. I use a normal saline solution because it's ionized from the salt content. It's amazing how fast these patients come back. They begin feeling better just on that alone because they have been chronically dehydrated forever.

Good hydration is only one factor required to remove water-soluble toxins through the urine, bile, and stool. Our kidneys, liver, and bowels must also be in good working order to eliminate these toxins. Keeping the liver in tip-top shape is important because it removes harmful fat-soluble toxins in a two-step enzymatic process, known as phase I and phase II detoxification (biotransformation). Specific reactions help to break down these fat-soluble toxins into safe, non-toxic, water-soluble compounds, which are then flushed out through the kidneys or colon.

Nutrition plays a significant role for these reactions to function optimally. This is why whole organic foods are important. The nutrients needed in phase I detoxification include, the B vitamins (B2, B3, B6, and B12), folic acid, glutathione, and flavonoids such as catechins, which are found in green tea. The nutrients needed in phase II detoxification include, methionine, cysteine, magnesium, glutathione, Vitamin B5, B12, Vitamin C, glycine, taurine, glutamine, folic acid, and choline. When either or both of these pathways is not functioning properly, toxins will pass through the liver unaffected, moving into the bloodstream, where they are deposited into various body tissues to add to your total body burden.

Good digestive health is needed, not only to promote nutrient absorption from food but for the elimination of toxins once they have been biotransformed. Having a digestive system burdened with constipation, chronic diarrhea, food allergies, inflammatory bowel diseases (such as Crohn's disease or ulcerative colitis), malabsorption syndromes (such as celiac disease, which decreases the ability of the digestive tract to digest and absorb nutrients from food), and lack of digestive enzymes or stomach acid will disrupt elimination and lead to re-absorption of these toxins back into your body.

The body burden of these toxins will eventually manifest in a constellation of signs and symptoms seemingly unrelated but having an impaired digestive system as the common denominator. (See Table 8.4)

Life as You Know it Must End

I've been working with a lady who is struggling with breast cancer. Every time she goes back to the doctor for chemotherapy, they do more testing. The results show a steady increase in the cancer of her breast, she only has one now, and I've told her, "Listen: life as you know it has to end if you want to get well."

That means she has to avoid everything connected with environmental estrogens: all pesticides, cleaners, and other household products, and every possible toxin. I instructed her to start using baking soda and forget about using toothpaste and cosmetics, as all of them have estrogen in their eyeliners and makeup. "You have to start using more natural products," I told her, recommending that she switch to a natural shampoo and even take a good look at her vitamins.

The vitamins manufactured by the big pharmaceutical companies are still synthetic. You have to take a whole-food-based vitamin for it to be healthful. Even then, you are isolating the vitamin from the enzymes, cofactors, and other good things that make natural, whole foods so nourishing for the body.

Trying to extract all that and put it into one pill, even though it's better than doing nothing, is not as good as following a healthy diet.

"You need to install a household water filtration system to remove the chlorine and other impurities coming through your household pipes, and you need a charcoal filter even when you are taking a shower," I said. She also can't have drapes and can't use plastics. She has to eliminate all sources of toxins.

The point is that, for her, she has no margin of error if she wants to turn the cancer around and save her life. We, who don't have cancer, can afford a little bit more of a margin than she can. But only as long as our immune systems are working well and we've chosen to support this with healthy-living practices, including a low-stress lifestyle, positive mental attitude, high-quality diet, and bioidentical hormone therapy. Otherwise, life as we know it also must come to an end.

Table 8.1: Chemicals in popular fragrances

Popular fragrances contain 14 secret chemicals on average

Chemicals found in lab tests but not listed on product labels

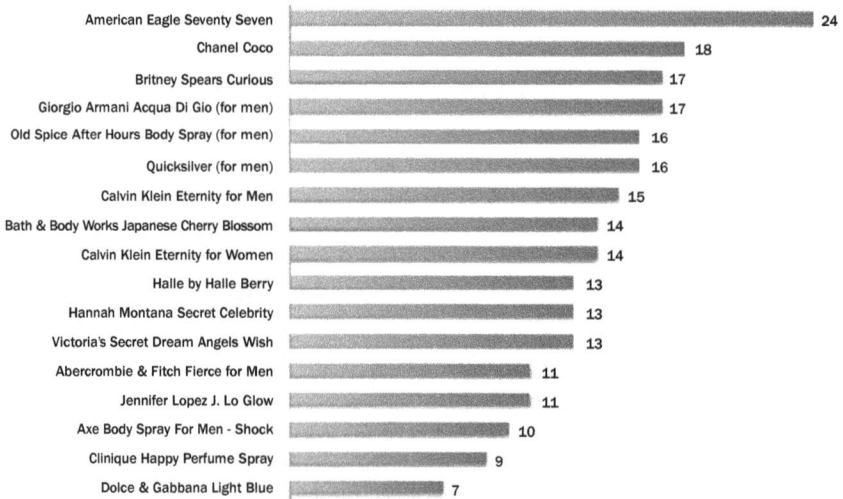

American Eagle Seventy Seven	24
Chanel Coco	18
Britney Spears Curious	17
Giorgio Armani Acqua Di Gio (for men)	17
Old Spice After Hours Body Spray (for men)	16
Quicksilver (for men)	16
Calvin Klein Eternity for Men	15
Bath & Body Works Japanese Cherry Blossom	14
Calvin Klein Eternity for Women	14
Halle by Halle Berry	13
Hannah Montana Secret Celebrity	13
Victoria's Secret Dream Angels Wish	13
Abercrombie & Fitch Fierce for Men	11
Jennifer Lopez J. Lo Glow	11
Axe Body Spray For Men - Shock	10
Clinique Happy Perfume Spray	9
Dolce & Gabbana Light Blue	7

Source: Environmental Working Group analysis of product labels and tests commissioned by the Campaign for Safe Cosmetics. Health risks from secret chemicals depend on the mixture in each product, the chemicals' hazards, the amounts that absorb into the body, and individual vulnerability to health problems.

Table 8.2: Chemical sensitizers in popular perfumes, colognes, and body sprays

	TOTAL SENSITIZING CHEMICALS	ALPHA-ISOMETHYL IONONE	AMYLCINNAMALDEHYDE	BENZYL ALCOHOL	BENZYL BENZOATE	BENZYL CINNAMATE	BENZYL SALICYLATE	CINNAMAL	CINNAMYL ALCOHOL	CITRAL	CITRONELLOL	COUMARIN	EUGENOL	EVERNIA FURFURACEA EXTRACT	FARNESOL	GERANIOL	HEXYL CINNAMAL	HYDROXYCITRONELLAL	ISOEUGENOL	LILIAL	LIMONENE	LINALOOL	LYRAL	LINALYL ACETATE	LINALYL ANTHRANILATE
Giorgio Armani Acqua Di Gio	19	•	•	•	•	•	•	•		•	•	•		•		•	•	•	•	•	•	•		•	•
Jennifer Lopez J. Lo Glow	16	•		•	•		•		•		•		•		•	•	•	•		•	•	•	•		•
Calvin Klein Eternity for Women	15		•	•		•		•		•		•				•		•	•	•	•	•	•	•	
Bath & Body Works Japanese Cherry Blossom	13	•		•		•	•	•		•	•	•			•			•	•			•	•		
Britney Spears Curious	13	•		•		•		•	•		•		•	•	•	•	•	•			•	•		
Calvin Klein Eternity for Men	13		•					•	•	•		•		•	•		•			•	•	•	•	•	•
Quicksilver for Men	13	•			•		•	•	•		•	•		•	•				•	•	•		•	•
Victoria's Secret Dream Angels Wish	13	•			•		•		•		•	•	•			•		•	•	•	•	•	•
Chanel Coco	12			•		•	•	•		•	•		•	•	•	•	•	•
Clinique Happy	10	•		•			•	•		•	•	•	•	•
Halle by Halle Berry	9			•		•	•		•		•	•	•	•
Abercrombie & Fitch Fierce	8				•	•	•		•		•	•	•
American Eagle Seventy Seven	7				•			•		•	•	•	•	•
Hannah Montana Secret Celebrity	5	•				•		•	•	•
Dolce & Gabbana Light Blue	4				•	•		•	•
Old Spice After Hours Body Spray	4					•	•	•	•
AXE Bodyspray For Men Shock	3					•	•	•

• Sensitizing chemical listed on ingredient label or found in product testing. Some of these chemicals such as eugenol. lllal or limonene, were listed on some but not all product labels, while others, such as linalool derivatives linalyl acetate and linalyl anthranilate, were not listed on any product label.

Source EWG analysis of product labels and rate commissioned by the Campaign for Safe Cosmetics.

Table 8.3: Hormone-disrupting chemicals in popular perfumes, colognes, and body sprays

	Total hormone disrupting chemicals	BENZOPHENONE-1	BENZOPHENONE-2	BENZYL BENZOATE	BENZYL SALICYLATE	BHT	DIETHYL PHTHAULATE	GALAXOLIDE	LILIAL	MUSK KETONE	OCTINOXATE	OXYBENZONE
Halle by Halle Berry	7			•		•	•	•	•		•	•
Quicksilver	7				•	•	•		•	•	•	
Jennifer Lopez J. Lo Glow	7			•	•	•	•	•	•			
American Eagle Seventy Seven	6			•			•	•	•		•	
Bath & Body Works Japanese Cherry Blossom	6			•	•	•		•	•		•	
Calvin Klein Eternity (for women)	6		•	•	•		•	•	•			
Calvin Klein Eternity for Men	5						•	•	•		•	
Chanel Coco	5				•		•	•	•		•	
Giorgio Armani Acqua Di Gio	5	•		•	•	•		•	•			
Vicoria's Secret Dream Angels Wish	4				•		•	•	•			
Britney Spears Curious	4			•	•		•	•				
Clinique Happy	3						•	•	•			
Hannah Montana Secret Celebrity	3						•	•			•	
Dolce & Gabbana Light Blue	3					•		•			•	
Old Spice After Hours Body Spray	2						•	•				
Abercrombie & Finch Fierce	1						•					
AXE Bodyspray for Men - Shock	1							•				

• Detected in product testing or listed in ingredient label
Source EWG analysis of product labels and rate commissioned by the Campaign for Safe Cosmetics, and results of hormones system studies in the literature.

Table 8.4   Signs that an Impaired Detoxification Capacity

Digestion, elimination problems (constipation, bloating, diarrhea, nausea, heartburn)	
Elevated cholesterol	Blood sugar and hormonal balance
Overweight/underweight	PMS
Allergies	Asthma
Skin Disorders	Frequent Flus, Colds, Sinus Infections
Fatigue	Muscle and Joint Pain, Fibromyalgia
Anger, Depression, Irritability	Anger, Depression, Irritability
Dark Circles Under Eyes	Chemical Sensitivities

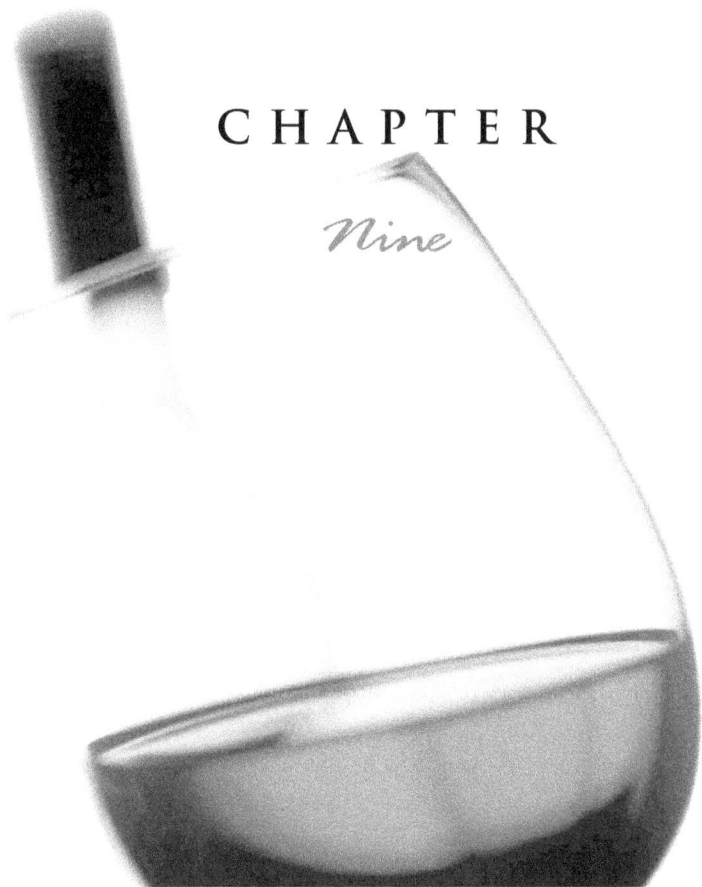

CHAPTER

Nine

CHAPTER NINE

Your Own Worst Enemy

"Progress is impossible without change, and those who cannot change their minds, cannot change anything."

G e o r g e   B e r n a r d   S h a w

Nature is coded for survival, but until recently it was usually the physically strong that survived. Now we are dying of affluence: too much unhealthy food and not enough need to keep physically fit and strong. Add to this the toxic habits we indulge in and the result is the 20th century diseases that are killing us today.

Although you may have a genetic predisposition toward coronary artery disease, heart attack, cancer, or whatever fearful way in which you expect to travel the same road as your parents, it doesn't mean that you are going to get it. Through the emerging science of epigenetics, we know that cells are not irreversibly programmed for the diseases in your family; a genetic disposition is only 25 percent (at most) of the equation and it is possible to reverse this through the choices you make.

Right now, if your father died of a heart attack at the age of 50 and you're smoking, not exercising, and eating fast food or engaging in other unhealthy indulgences, you're also likely to have a heart attack, and probably around the age of 50. But if you work to overwhelm that genetic predisposition and change the expression of those genes by the way you are living now, you won't be doomed to this dismal fate.

The most important factors are how you think, what nutrition you have, and the lifestyle you follow, including your willingness to turn away from unhealthy habits. You can create a new cycle of positivity and overwhelm that ability to create disease.

We are bombarded and inflamed daily with free radicals, which causes metabolic inflammation leading to heart disease, arthritis, diabetes, and other ailments of aging. They are the result of poor diet, imbalanced hormones, exposure to toxins, and lack of exercise. If you also make unwise choices like smoking—there are a trillion free radicals in one cigarette!—your chances of getting sick with something like cancer will skyrocket.

You didn't start out being your own worst enemy. But now the quality of the rest of your days depends on starting right now to change, such as eliminating unhealthy habits and addressing long-standing heath issues. Eating better, getting more exercise, and guarding your health all have lifelong implications in terms of disease expression.

Sick of Smoking

If you are a smoker, you likely acquired this addiction early in your childhood, either in your home or through your social group. If your parents smoked, the chances of you not smoking are low because kids like to do what their parents do. Or you may have been pressured into smoking by the need to be included among your peers.

Every addiction has a social as well as physical component. The desire to appear "grown up" tempted many of us to start smoking. Think of all the old movies and advertising that portrayed smoking as glamorous and socially acceptable. That doesn't happen today, but it was very common to find those depictions in earlier decades.

Children often learn this extremely bad habit by inhaling it from their parents, and we now know that second-hand smoke is equally detrimental to health. I have heard about and known people, dying of lung cancer, who never smoked. They lived or worked in offices where people used to smoke and this is almost as bad.

The offspring of smokers are very sick children. They develop asthma, get more bronchitis, and are primed to adopt this unhealthy addiction through years of childhood exposure to it. Their parents, because of the nature of this addiction, find it difficult to break. So one thing they tell me is, "Listen, I go outside to smoke." I always have to tell them, "I can smell you from ten feet away. Your child can, too. Have you ever heard of third-hand smoke? You go outside to smoke, then come back inside and sit on the furniture. You hold your children and they breathe the residue of your smoking into their lungs from your furniture and your clothing. So it's almost as bad."

Recent research describes health hazards may occur simply by touching a surface that has been contaminated with tobacco smoke, such as clothing or furnishings. Lawrence Berkeley National Laboratory in Calfornia discovered that nicotine reacts with a common indoor air pollutant found in smokers' homes and cars, which is called nitrous acid, and forms carcinogenic compounds known as tobacco-specific nitrosamines (TSNAs). TSNAs were found to persist hours after the cigarette smoke has cleared. According to the authors, "These findings raise concerns about exposures to the tobacco smoke residue that has been recently dubbed 'third-hand smoke' ". They urged particular caution should be exercised to reduce the exposure of infants and young children to these toxins.

You must find a way to stop! If not for you, then do it for your children and grandchildren. Exposure to cigarette smoke as infants and toddlers has long-term consequences for their health. These children will show permanent lung damage as young adults, despite never having smoked.

In addition, you're already being exposed to numerous toxins in your environment. You have to avoid what I call the landmines, and the biggest one is smoking. It leads to the whole stress cycle that I've described in previous chapters.

Smoking dramatically increases the free radicals in your body from arsenic and other poisons in the smoke itself. When you inhale all that, it causes a lot of free-radical damage in your lungs, leading to emphysema. It creates peripheral vascular disease, where the blood vessels narrow all over your body, and the reduction of blood in your lower extremities means that you have pain when you walk. It can close off an artery in your brain, which means that you'll have a stroke or heart attack.

A lot of men who smoke have erection problems. Narrowing of small blood vessels includes the ones going to the penis, and these guys can't have erections. When I see them in the office, the first thing they have to do is get off smoking. They will still have damage but some of it can be reversed.

I always say the skin is a reflection of the inside of the body. If you have very good skin, you probably have very good insides. Smoking leads to free-radical-associated loss of collagen and elastin. It interferes with your body's mechanism for breaking down old skin and renewing it, leading to the development of age spots, wrinkles, and white heads. It causes more skin damage that any other environmental factor and can make you look very unpleasant.

I use a very shocking slide of female twins in my esthetic practice. One had smoked from the age of 20; one did not. At the age of 55, the difference in their appearance is unbelievable. The one who smoked looks about 80 and the one who did not looks to be about 40. It ages you that much.

The damage is system wide. Hormonally, it affects the thyroid, testicles, ovaries, adrenals, and pituitary. It leads to roughening of the entire body and less overall efficiency. We have enough exposure to toxins in our environment; why are you stepping on your own self-made landmine?

Yo-Yo Dieting

The thyroid is your metabolic engine, determining what your base metabolic rate will be. Crash diets cause a biologically-programmed interruption in its functioning that actually results in weight gain. Along the way, hormones and other metabolic processes are disrupted.

The thyroid is stimulated to make its hormones in the following proportions: 80 percent of T4, which is ultimately converted to T3 in the bloodstream, and 20 percent of T3, which is the active thyroid. But in a physiological response that likely dates back to early Paleolithic man and conditions of starvation, T4 can also be converted into a reversed form of T3 that is not metabolically active and has the effect of shutting down your basal metabolic rate. When there isn't a lot of food, the thyroid makes this reversed version of T3.

It happens when you are doing a lot of crash dieting because the body sees this as as a sign of scarcity. So it slows everything down; no matter what you do you're not going to lose weight. With a lot of up-and-down, yo-yo dieting, you will permanently lower your basal metabolic rate. It will stay on neutral and you will actually gain weight on fewer calories. Rather than gaining weight on ten calories, you will gain weight on one calorie.

So crash dieting, whether you are following a program that's low-carb, high protein, high vegetable, or whatever, it all results in this problem. It's truly a yo-yo because as soon as you quit the severe restrictions of whatever diet you're following, all the weight comes back again; it's only a short-term solution. This same mechanism occurs in people under increased stress. Increased stress results in increased cortisol, which interferes with the conversion of T4 to active T3 and results in more reverse T3 is made. This slows down the metabolism and leads to stress-induced weight gain.

Diets also tend to utilize artificial sweeteners as a way of curbing a sweet tooth. A recent 11-year study from the Bringham Women's Hospital in Boston, MA, conducted on 3000 women, indicated that drinking two or more artificially sweetened beverages a day doubled the risk of experiencing unnaturally rapid kidney-function deterioration. Sodium intake was implicated as the cause; diet beverages contain excessive amounts of sodium, higher than sugared drinks and harmful chemical sweeteners.

Stevia is a much better alternative than artificial sweeteners and one of my favorites. This herb from South America is up to 300 times sweeter than sugar. In the United States, the FDA recently added it to their "generally regarded as safe" list last year. This designation means that a chemical or substance added to food is considered safe by experts, and so is exempt from the food-additive tolerance requirements listed in the *Federal Food, Drug, and Cosmetic Act* . Available as a greenish powder, stevia imparts a powerful sweetness with an herbal undertone.

There are other natural sweeteners, all of which reduce detrimental blood-sugar spikes with ingestion, because the nutrients and minerals found in whole-food sugars help with their metabolism. Annie Berthold-Bond and Nava Atlas, authors of *The Vegetarian 5-Ingredient Gourmet*, discuss this and offer a list of less-refined sweeteners. They include agave nectar, barley malt, honey, maltose, maple sugar, molasses, sorghum syrup, and sucanat among others (see Table 9.1).

Table 9.1: Sweetener Equivalents for One-Half Cup of Sugar (From The Vegetarian 5-Ingredient Gourmet)
Barley malt: 1 1/2 cup
Date sugar: 1 cup
Fruit juice concentrate: equal to sugar
Granular fruit sweeteners: equal to sugar
Honey: 1/3 cup
Maltose (from sprouted grains): 1 1/4 cup
Maple syrup: equal to sugar
Molasses: 1/3 cup
Rice syrup: 1 1/4 cup
Sorghum syrup: 1/3 cup
Sucanat: equal to sugar
Organic sugar: equal to sugar

The health-damaging evidence is stacking up against chemical products such as aspartame and sucralose. In the 1980s, aspartame (found in products such as NutraSweet, Equal, Spoonful, Benevia, and Equal-Measure) was found to cause cancer in laboratory rats. The ingredients in aspartame include aspartic acid, phenylalanine, and methyl alcohol, all of which are toxic.

Aspartic acid, which comprises 40 percent of aspartame, is one of a class of amino acids known as excitotoxins, which means this brain neurotransmitter will "excite" your brain cells to death. It allows a large influx of calcium into your brain cells, activating free radicals that kill the cells. Supplements that offer natural protection against these excitotoxins include magnesium, ginkgo biloba, omega-3 fatty acids, selenium, red clover, and zinc.

Phenylalanine, which comprises 50 percent of aspartame, lowers the body's seizure threshold and depletes serotonin (the "feel good" neurotransmitter), causing manic depression, panic attacks, rage, and violence. In people with phenylketonuria, it is particularly unsafe because this congenital condition (which afflicts over 15,000 Americans), involves an enzyme disorder that inhibits the metabolism of phenylalanine that could result in brain damage. Methyl alcohol (wood alcohol) comprises 10 percent of aspartame; this chemical converts within your body into formaldehyde (embalming fluid) and then into formic acid (ant-sting poison). These two metabolites both lead to immune and nervous-system dysfunction. Drinking even one diet cola a day can cause a form of formaldehyde to build up in your cells. Diketopiperazine, a byproduct of aspartame metabolism, has been implicated in the occurrence of brain tumors.

Jean Carpers's book, *Food: Your Miracle Medicine,* reported that aspartame increases migraine frequency in more than 50 percent of the migraine patients participating in a study. Scientists believe it exacerbates depression and causes migraines by lowering serotonin levels. If you suffer these kinds of illnesses, you may want to consume foods that raise the level of serotonin in your brain.

A study published in the January 2008 issue of the *Journal of Toxicology and Environmental Health* revealed that a newer artificial sweetener, sucralose, alters gut microflora and inhibits the absorption of dietary nutrients. Marketed as being "made from sugar," it has undergone no long-term human studies to verify its safety. However, as with aspartame, initial studies revealed negative reactions in lab animals on which it was tested, indicating the possibility of similar problems in humans.

We have a lot of concerns related to food. In addition to contamination from pesticides, herbicides, and fungicides, genetically-modified foods and non-nutritious, processed "cardboard food" (as I like to call it) are just a few of the issues threatening out health. Additives are another problem: there are more than 3000 preservatives, flavorings, colors, and other ingredients added to food in the United States. The average American will eat their weight in food additives every year. Most are harmless but some may not be.

Food additives are substances added in small amounts to our food for specific purposes. There are generally five main reasons why chemicals are added to our foods. They include:

1.   Improving shelf life or storage time. Preservatives such as propylene glycol, a commonly used humectant, prevent food from drying out. Other preservatives, such as potassium sorbate, inhibit food spoilage due to microorganisms.

2.   Making food convenient and easy to prepare.

3.   Increasing the nutritional value. Vitamins and minerals are sometimes added to improve a food item's nutritional content; we see this in fortification programs such as adding iodine to salt.

4.   Improving the flavour of food.

5.   Enhancing the attractiveness of food products to improve customer acceptance. Many food colorings are added to replace colors lost during preparation or enhance the product's attractiveness. Natural pigments include annatto, beta-carotene, turmeric, and beet juice. But there are also a number of blue, red, and yellow artificial coloring agents, some of which have been linked to allergic reactions and possibly cancer.

As part of your program to age to perfection, you should educate yourself and be aware of detrimental food additives in your diet and consider avoiding them on any regular basis. You must make a decision to cut these out altogether, or at least start by eating fewer of them. Dr. Elson M. Hass, author of *Staying Healthy Shopper's Guide: Feed Your Family Safely*, describes 12 key additives to avoid and their health risks:

1.   Hydrogenated fats: These are mostly man-made fats used in bakery items and stick margarine. Avoid buying cookies, crackers, baked goods, or anything else that has hydrogenated oil on the ingredient list. These trans fats are proven to cause heart disease (they raise bad cholesterol (LDL) and lower good cholesterol (HDL)) and make conditions perfect for stroke, heart attacks, kidney failure, and limb loss due to vascular disease. Experts recommend that we consume no more than two grams of trans fats per day. This is near the recommendation by the AHA that no more than one percent of your total daily calories be from trans fat (based on a 2000 calorie per day diet).

2.   Artificial food colors: Derived from coal tar, 13 synthetic colorants have been banned by the FDA since 1956 because of public health concerns. Blue No. 1 and No. 2 are found in beverages, candy, baked goods, and pet food. They are considered low risk but have been linked to cancer in mice. Red No. 3, banned in cosmetics, is still used in dye cherries, fruit cocktail, candy, and baked goods and has shown to cause thyroid tumors in rats. Green No. 3, added to candy and beverages (rarely used), has been linked to bladder cancer. Widely used yellow No. 6, added to beverages, sausage, gelatin, baked goods, and candy, has been linked to tumors of the adrenal gland and kidney. Yellow No. 5 must be individually listed on ingredient labels, rather than referred to as artificial color, because it is associated with allergic reactions such as hives, runny nose, and shortness of breath.

3.   Nitrites and nitrates: These additives are added to bacon, ham, hot dogs, luncheon meats, smoked fish, and corned beef to stabilize the red color and add flavor. They aren't carcinogenic by themselves, but when they pair with chemicals called amines (which occur when cooked at high temperatures such as frying bacon or roasting ham), they become a potent cancer-causing chemical known as nitrosamine. When you eat foods containing nitrates, have a glass of orange juice at the same time (for instance, orange juice with your morning bacon). Vitamin C is known to inhibit the conversion to nitrosamines in your stomach.

4.   Sulfites (sulfur dioxide, metabisulfites, potassium metasulfite, and others): These are found naturally in beer and wine but they are also synthetically produced to reduce discoloration in dried fruit, dehydrated soup mixes, processed seafood, and syrups. They can cause reactions ranging from hives to death in many Americans.

5.   Sugar and sweeteners: Although non-toxic, too many Americans are consuming more than 30 to 40 percent of their daily calories from simple sugars (it should be no more than 10 percent). As a result, this excessive sugar intake has led to obesity, diabetes, and increased blood fats (increased triglycerides), and replaces good nutrition. Also, ingesting so many calories from sugar robs your body of valuable vitamins and minerals, as your body uses up these nutrients to metabolize sugar.

6.   Artifical sweeteners (aspartame, acesulfame K, and saccharin): See section above on aspartame. Saccharin (found in Sweet 'N Low) has been demonstrated to cause cancer in lab animals and is classified by the FDA as a weak carcinogen. Acesulfame-K (sold as Sweet One or Sunette, and found in chewing gum, instant coffee and tea, puddings, gelatin desserts, and nondairy creamers) has a chemical structure similar to saccharin and has promoted tumor growth in laboratory animals.

7.   MSG (monosodium glutamate): This is an amino acid used as a flavor enhancer in soups, salad dressing, chips, frozen entrees, and restaurant food. MSG can cause allergic and behavioral reactions, including headaches, dizziness, chest pains, depression, and mood swings. It has been described as a possible neurotoxin.

8.   Preservatives (butylated hydroxyanisole (BHA) and butylated hydroxytoluene (BHT), propyl gallate): BHA and BHT are chemical substances used to keep fats and oils from going rancid. They are found in cereals (from Total to Quaker Instant Oatmeal), chewing gum, potato chips, and vegetable oils. Studies have show them to increase the risk of cancer, accumulate in body tissues, cause liver enlargement, and retard the rate of DNA synthesis. Propyl gallate is often used in conjunction with BHA and BHT. It is found in meat products, chicken soup base, and chewing gum. Studies done in animals have suggested a link to cancer.

9.   Artificial flavors: They have been linked to allergic or behavioral reactions.

10.   Refined flour: They contain low nutrient calories and lead to altered insulin production.

11.   Salt (excessive): Although the body needs salt, excessive amounts can be dangerous to your health as it affects cardiovascular function, leading to high blood pressure, heart attack, stroke, or kidney failure.

12.   Olestra (artificial fat): This synthetic fat, known under the brand name Olean and found in some brands of potato chips, prevents

fats from being absorbed in your digestive system. This can lead to severe diarrhea, abdominal cramps, and gas. Unfortunately, it will also block healthy vitamin absorption (A, D, E, and K) from fat-soluble carotenoids that are found in fruits and vegetables.

Getting Over Overeating

At school, many of us weren't taught about good health habits, such as the benefits of exercise. Our schools are getting better at teaching students about healthy living, but they were also the source of some very bad habits laid down from early childhood. For example, there used to be soft drink and candy vending machines in schools, which encouraged kids to become addicted to products made from high-fructose corn syrup (HFCS). This chemical additive and preservative will increase the set-point for satiety; you literally won't realize when you're full.

The body processes the fructose in HFCS differently than it does old-fashioned cane or beet sugar, which in turn alters the way that metabolic-regulating hormones function. Unlike other types of carbohydrates made from glucose, HFCS does not stimulate the pancreas to produce insulin. It also leads to leptin resistance; this hormone is produced by the body's fat cells as weight is gained. It signals the brain that there are adequate energy (fat) stores and that it should stimulate the metabolism again. Both these hormones act as signals to the brain to turn down the appetite and control body weight.

In addition, HFCS does not appear to suppress the production of ghrelin, a hormone that increases hunger and appetite. A diet that is high in fructose will lead to consuming more calories. It also forces the liver to more readily convert fructose to fat in the bloodstream, in the form of triglycerides.

The end result is that our bodies are essentially tricked into wanting to eat more and, at the same time, store more fat. HFCS has promoted obesity and a lifelong addiction to sugary foods. If you are currently struggling with overeating, this toxin is a primary reason. As with any addiction, it causes cravings that are very difficult to control.

In addition, eating highly acidic foods creates more fat cells in your body. These cells are designed to take that acid away from your organs and isolate it where your body can't be harmed, but then things really get out of hand. Obesity leads to a functional hypothyroid problem and tremendous pressure on your adrenals to cope with all that sugar. Hormones are created within the fat; they cause your body's delicate balance to spiral out of control.

If you also have a habit of consuming chemical-laden fast foods loaded with trans-fatty acids, there is no wonder you feel bad and can't get better. The result is depression, lethargy, and cravings for foods you know you shouldn't eat. You comfort yourself, because you feel terrible, by eating more unhealthy food. You become the victim of your physiology: too tired to exercise and unable to stop eating the very foods that will eventually kill you.

This negative spiral leads to serious health problems such as Type II diabetes. Chronic disease is the legacy of consuming addictive substances. There may be comfort in knowing that it originally wasn't your fault. But not stopping this unhealthy pattern is now your responsibility.

You must get your diet under control. A good place to start is by eating complex carbohydrates. As I discussed in chapter 4, the fiber in whole-grain foods slows down the digestion process; this keeps your insulin levels under control. They will give you a feeling of satiety, reduce cravings, sustain better levels of energy, and help you to eliminate toxins.

Simple carbohydrates are highly processed foods; they are usually loaded with high-fructose corn syrup. These are high-glycemic foods and it's the insulin spike from eating them that causes so much damage. It doesn't happen overnight. It takes years.

The cumulative effect of unhealthy trans fat, chemical additives, and the relentless spiking of sugar and insulin makes the difference between living well into your nineties and beyond or having a heart attack in your fifties.

You have to start somewhere to lose weight and change your eating habits. Bioidentical hormone therapy is one way to support your body in shedding the pounds. Anything you do to try to improve metabolism and physical functioning will help you to lose weight, and bioidentical hormone therapy does exactly that. It supports all of your body's physiological processes.

It creates a positive cascade. With hormonal support you start feeling better and have more energy; this supports your motivation to achieve your weight-loss goals by adopting a fitness program to further ramp up your metabolism. As the pounds come off, you feel even healthier, which naturally increases your willpower. Every little thing you do becomes magnified in the body because inflammation is reduced throughout your body.

The important thing is to start. Eventually, you will lose weight, you'll living better, your depression begins to lift, and you'll enjoy an upscale cycle. It encourages you to go further in terms of improving your health.

Gateway to the Body

The mouth is the gateway to the body and a marker of health as many chronic diseases have an oral connection. It was Charles Mayo (co-founder of the Mayo Clinic) who noted over 90 years ago that people who keep their teeth live an average of ten years longer than people who do not. Even former Surgeon General Donna Shalala said in her 2000 address, "The terms oral health and general health should not be interpreted as separate entities. Oral health is integral to general health."

How we take care of our teeth, gums, and mouth has much to do with how healthy we age. For example, taking care of our teeth will ensure that we keep them for life. And keeping our teeth and gums healthy contributes to aging to perfection since, without them, we cannot chew or bite the hardy fruits and vegetables that will keep us healthy.

The human mouth is home to billions of bacteria with more than 100 species of bacteria, as well as hundreds of species of fungi, protozoa, and viruses. It has more microorganisms than any other part of the body except the intestines. Many are constantly seeking to invade more deeply into our tissues by way of our 32 teeth with their deep mucosal penetration. Poor oral hygiene will lead to a low-grade inflammation of the gums (gingivitis), which is caused by bacteria and dental plaque that create a biofilm that stimulates an immune response in the soft tissues surrounding the teeth. The gums then become inflamed and irritated, appearing swollen, red, and bleed easily. This plaque cannot be removed by the body's natural immune response and must be mechanically removed.

Left untreated, this infection and inflammation will extend to the gums and bone supporting the teeth (periodontitis), which will have detrimental effects both locally and throughout the body. Locally, periodontal disease will cause loss of periodontal tissue, pocket formation, and loosening and loss of teeth. Systemically, anaerobic bacteria discharge hydrogen sulfide, ammonia, amines, and toxins that serve as inflammatory mediators throughout the body. These bacteria and their byproducts enter the circulation, stimulating the liver and white blood cells to increase their production of inflammatory proteins such as C-reactive protein, inflammatory cytokines (IL-1 beta, tumor necrosis factor-alpha, and IL-6), blood coagulation and adhesion factors, and increased blood lipid levels.

This inflammatory cascade has been implicated in the increased risk of developing systemic diseases such as diabetes (increases in C-reactive protein cause fat cells (adipocytes) to store more fat and burn less energy), causing the initiation and progression of atherosclerosis (bacteria have been recovered from atherosclerotic plaques and major arteries), which leads to heart attacks and strokes. Research confirms that periodontitis is an independent risk factor for heart attacks and strokes with the degree of risk higher for stroke than for heart attacks. The more teeth that are affected by periodontal disease, the higher the risk. The onset of dementia has also been implicated from periodontal inflammation that causes increasing atherosclerosis. The treatment of periodontal disease will result in reduction of serum inflammatory markers and improved levels of glycated hemoglobin, a measure of long-term glucose control.

In addition, researchers have found that pregnant women with periodontitis were 7.5 times more likely to have a preterm low-birth-weight infant than unaffected pregnant women. Thus, oral health care must be included in any comprehensive prenatal health care program.

The World Health Organization considers poor oral hygiene a risk factor in the development of cardiovascular disease, diabetes mellitus, cancer, and chronic respiratory diseases. Researchers from *Lancet Oncology* studied 48,000 men over 18 years and found that periodontal disease was associated with a "small but significant increase in overall cancer risk, which persisted in never-smokers." The research team also found significant associations between oral health status and lung, kidney, blood, and pancreatic cancers. Researchers at the Harvard School of Public Health also concluded that periodontitis is associated with an increased risk of pancreatic cancer.

Like osteopenia and osteoporosis, estrogen deficiency is also a risk factor for periodontal disease. Women using hormone replacement demonstrated decreased indicators of gingivitis and periodontitis severity compared to estrogen-deficit females.

In people with periodontal disease, scientists have found that bacteria that grow in the oral cavity can be aspirated into the lung to cause respiratory diseases such as pneumonia. In fact, one study found a fivefold increase in chronic respiratory disease in subjects that had poor oral hygiene when compared to those with good oral hygiene. Periodontal bacteria have been cultured from infected lung fluids and lung tissues.

We know that lifestyle factors always have an influence in the success or failure of many therapies. Smoking, stress, depression, and alcohol consumption are risk factors for periodontitis. However, good nutrition and exercise in the form of walking has been shown to benefit periodontal health. Several nutrients have also been demonstrated to help with periodontal health as part of an oral hygiene program. Among these are coenzyme Q 10, green tea, aloe vera, and pomegranate. Other beneficial ingredients for healthy teeth and gums include xylitol, lactoferrin, and folic acid.

Two Kinds of Drinking

When it comes to caffeine and wine consumption, it is an issue of excess and not of ingestion. A little bit is beneficial; too much is bad for your health.

Moderate amounts of caffeine, no more than two cups a day of tea or coffee gives you the antioxidant benefit of polyphenols. These inflammation fighters are found in tea, coffee, and chocolate. In addition, since drinking coffee or tea is dehydrating (caffeine is a diuretic), you must ensure that you also drink an equivalent amount of water (on top of the quantities needed for proper hydration; see chapter 7 for a discussion).

Of course, caffeine helps your alertness. The polyphenols in caffeine cause a small elevation of dopamine levels in your brain, which is a mood enhancer and gives you a feeling of pleasure in your body. Researchers at Harvard

University (Cambridge, MA) also found that coffee reduces the risk of diabetes. *Archives of Internal Medicine* reported a review of 18 studies involving almost 500,000 people indicating that up to four cups of decaffeinated coffee or tea daily reduces the incidence of Type II diabetes by up to 30 percent.

Athletes have known for more than 60 years that caffeine before a competition improves both speed and endurance. It increases the amount of sugar their muscles use for energy. Sugar requires less oxygen than fat to be converted to energy. Caffeine can lower the risk of diabetes by the same mechanism: driving sugar from the blood into muscles, thus lowering blood-sugar levels. Other components in coffee such as ligans and chlorogenic acids (a family of esters) may help prevent diabetes by their antioxidant effects.

While hard liquor is never good for you, red wine is a very rich source of reservatrol, another antioxidant polyphenol. The skins of wine grapes have high concentrations of reservatrol. Depending on your body's ability to metabolize it, one or two glasses of wine a day will offer these benefits; more than this, however, will affect your liver.

There are 72 different detoxification enzymes in the liver, and alcohol affects every one of them. If your liver is functioning to detoxify this alcohol, it won't be performing other vital actions. Too much alcohol can also destroy neurons in your brain.

One problem with beer is the hops, which are a source of estrogen. They inhibit production of testosterone. When I put men on bioidentical testosterone, I tell them not to drink very much beer because it counteracts the effect. If a man is not responding to bioidentical testosterone, getting him completely off alcohol will make the difference. After that, he can often work up gradually to one glass a day.

Too much exposure to the estrogen in beer is also not good for a woman unless her levels have dropped. Only occasional glasses of beer would be advisable, and if she is on bioidentical estrogen, she should not have beer at all.

Here Comes the Sun

Today's common medical advice about staying out of the sun and using sunscreens has contributed to a growing health concern, often called the "unrecognized silent epidemic," of Vitamin D deficiency. It is estimated that 70 to 80 percent of all Americans are deficient in this vitamin, particularly darker-skinned people, the elderly, children and teens, and breast-fed infants. I have found this proportion to be accurate in my practice.

This is particularly appalling since spending a little time outdoors, soaking up the ultraviolet rays (UV), is all it takes to get sufficient Vitamin D. In fact, the sun's power to heal has been known for centuries. Yet, today we are told to "stay out of the sun because it is harmful."

Of course, too much of any good thing can make you sick, and the sun is no different. Sunburn is probably cancer promoting, but no sun exposure can lead to the same thing. Being careful not to burn is important for good skin health. But this medical advice, to completely avoid the sun, has led to such a severe deficiency in so many people that it is implicated in numerous chronic disease conditions.

Studies show that the sun enhances health and longevity by stimulating the production of Vitamin D from your skin. This vitamin is critical because it regulates calcium and phosphorus metabolism and is involved in activating 10 percent of the human genome (your body's genetic code) more efficiently. It also decreases cancer by 50 to 60 percent overall. Its presence is needed for optimal performance of muscle function, immunology, neurology, cancer protection, and many other benefits. Vitamin D levels will fluctuate with geographical location, UV index, skin type, and exposure to the sun.

As seen in chapter 4, it is so important to monitor your Vitamin D levels using the 25-hydroxy D or calcidiol blood level (instead of the 1,25-hydroxy D or calcitriol level) to ensure adequate Vitamin D is available for optimum health. Your 25-hydroxylvitamin D levels should be in the range of 50 to 80 ng/ml. It is UVB radiation (of 280 to 315 nm) that stimulates the production of Vitamin D in the skin; it constitutes three to five percent of the total UV radiation that gets through the atmosphere. Due to its shorter wavelength, it only penetrates the outer skin layer, which can result in sunburn and the development of non-melanoma skin cancer such as squamous cell carcinoma. UVA radiation (315 to 400 nm), which constitutes 95 to 97 percent of total UV radiation, causes skin to pigment or tan. Its longer wavelength allows it to penetrate deeper into skin tissue, which is most responsible for generating free radicals that may damage DNA and skin cells.

Your adequate sun exposure will depend on the local UV index and your skin type (see Table 9.2). The UV index helps people to protect themselves from overexposure. It is an international standard measurement of UV radiation from the sun for a particular place and time. It predicts how strong UV intensity will be at the sun's highest point, which is two to four hours on either side of solar noon. You can find out what your local UV index is by accessing The Weather Channel (weather.com) or the EPA Sunwise Index (epa.gov/sunwise).

The closer you get to solar noon, the more UVB is available from sun exposure. Early in the day and late in the day, sunlight provides only UVA, which doesn't help you to make Vitamin D. But it can still cause skin damage, so you shouldn't expose your skin intentionally when the UVI is less than 3. To manufacture adequate levels of Vitamin D naturally, 50 to 75 percent of your skin must be exposed (such as shorts with a sleeveless shirt, or a swimsuit) to the sun between 10:30 a.m. and 2:00 p.m., about three to four times per week when your local UV index is 3 or higher.

Table 9.2: Sun Exposure Chart for Different Skin Types and UV Index					
Skin Type	UVI: 0-2	UVI: 3-5	UVI: 6-7	UVI: 8-10	UVI: 11+
Always burn, never tan	0 minutes	10-15 min	5-10 min	2-5 min	1-2 min
Easily burn, rarely tan	0 minutes	15-20 min	10-15 min	5-10 min	2-5 min
Occas. burn, slowly tan	0 minutes	20-30 min	20-15 min	10-15 min	5-10 min
Rarely burn, rapidly tan	0 minutes	30-40 min	20-30 min	15-20 min	10-15 min
Never burn, always dark	0 minutes	40-60 min	30-40 min	20-30 min	15-20 min

Regular, safe exposure to the sun is the best way to maintain optimal levels of Vitamin D. A spring-break-style, concentrated exposure for one week is just a recipe for sunburn and is ill advised given the potential for very negative, long-term skin consequences. Starting in early spring, if you follow a practice of gradually increasing daily exposure to the sun, you will acclimate your skin to its recurring intensity without the risk of detrimental sunburns.

For a light-skinned person, begin with sun exposure of your arms, legs, and trunk for 10 minutes a day at least three times per week, increasing to 20 minutes to two hours throughout the summer. A darker-skinned person should be outside for a significantly longer period of time (as much as ten times more exposure), depending on skin type.

A person over the age of 50 will need to double this sun exposure time. It is more difficult to synthesize Vitamin D as we age (a 70-year-old will produce 25 percent less Vitamin D than a 20-year old). Skin that is deeply tanned or genetically darker contains more melanin, which is the skin's natural pigment. It serves as an innate sunscreen, reducing penetration of the UVB radiation needed to make Vitamin D. Therefore, more time in the sun is needed in darker-skinned and older people to make sufficient amounts of Vitamin D.

If you live in northern climates or spend little time in the sun, you will need Vitamin D supplementation. Food can provide some of what you need, but your total consumption will probably average 200 to 400 IU per day, which is insufficient. As a result, you may need Vitamin D supplementation. The average American will need about 20 to 25 IU of Vitamin D per pound of body weight to get their levels up to the 50 to 80 ng/ml range. Ensure that you supplement with Vitamin D3 (cholecalciferol), not its inferior cousin, Vitamin D2 (ergocalciferol). Vitamin D3 is the form your body manufactures through exposure to the sun, and it is also found in natural food sources.

The healthy use of a tanning bed. Tanning beds can offer help with production of Vitamin D, but you must use them judiciously. Only expose your skin to the point that it turns the slightest pink color in Caucasian people. Avoid, at all costs, the risk of getting sunburned. The ratio of UVA to UVB light from the sun is 10:1 to 20:1. But some tanning bulbs can have a ratio as high as 100:1, which will be more likely to cause photoaging (wrinkles and age spots) and will not significantly enhance your health. You can optimize your production of Vitamin D by using a tanning bed that produces more UVB in proportion to UVA. So be sure to ask for the tanning bed with the highest UVB to UVA ratio.

Another problem with older tanning beds is the use of magnetic ballasts to generate the light, causing you to also be exposed to large amounts of harmful electromagnetic fields (EMF). EMFs are found in home appliances, computers, home wiring, and utility power lines. A 650-page report, released in August 2007 by the Bioinitative Working Group, demonstrated that chronic exposure to even low-level radiation (such as a cell phone) can cause a variety of cancers, impaired immunity, and can contribute to Alzheimer's disease, dementia, heart block, and many other health problems.

Called the *"BioInitiative Report: A Rationale for a Biologically-based Public Exposure Standard for Electromagnetic Fields* (ELF and RF)," it cited more than 2000 studies detailing the toxic effects of excessive EMF exposure. EMF radiation may be the reason, in addition to the higher UVA exposure, why the risk of melanoma increases by 75 percent for people who use tanning beds before the age of 35. To avoid this risk, you must only frequent tanning salons using more efficient, safer electronic ballasts.

A good diet can help to inhibit the development of skin cancer arising from moderate, natural sun exposure. This includes unprocessed vegetables and fruits with a good ratio of omega-6 fats to omega-3 fats (no higher than 3:1, and 1:1 is optimal). The antioxidants found in fruits and vegetables migrate to the skin and prevent the DNA damage that can lead to malignancies. These are more protective against sun-induced radiation damage, which can cause wrinkles and cancers, than any sunscreen. As Dr. John Cannell from the Vitamin D Council (vitamindcouncil.org) eloquently states:

"The people who get sunburned are modern humans who live and work indoors, avoid fruit and vegetables, love french fries and chips, hate salmon, and go to the beach two or three times in the summer to roast themselves. Frequent sunburns, especially in childhood, are but one factor in melanoma—genetics and diet are more important."

It is regular, controlled sun exposure, without sunburns, that significantly decreases the risk of melanoma and other diseases. Conversely, a poor diet with high omega-6 fats in proportion to omega-3 fats increases your risk.

When you are going to be out in the sun for an extended period of time, the best protection is a hat and shirt rather than relying exclusively on sunscreens. Even the International Agency for Research on Cancer (IARC) advocates wearing protective clothing, seeking shade, and timing outdoor play to avoid peak sun before using sunscreens. Other reasons to avoid sunscreen unless absolutely necessary include the following:

1. Contrary to traditional medical advice, most sunscreens actually increase your risk of disease by impeding your body's production of the valuable Vitamin D that keeps you healthy. An SPF 8 rated sunscreen will reduce its production by 97.5 percent; an SPF 15 rated sunscreen will reduce it by 99.9 percent.

2. There is controversy as to whether sunscreens actually prevent cancer. Many studies show that regular sunscreen use does reduce the risk of squamous cell carcinoma (only 16 percent of all skin cancers) but not other types of skin cancer, Melanoma, which accounts for only three to four percent of all skin cancers, is the deadliest, and is responsible for 75 percent of skin cancer deaths (basal cell carcinoma accounts for 80 percent of all skin cancers). In many studies, the use of sunscreen seems to contribute to the development of melanoma. No one knows the cause, but scientists speculate that sunscreen users stay out in the sun longer and wear less protective clothing with more overall radiation absorption, and free radicals released in the skin when sunscreen ingredients break down in sunlight contribute to its development. In addition, early generation sunscreens did not provide adequate UVA protection but did block UVB. There is still controversy around how much UVA and UVB actually contribute to the development of melanoma. This means that, when using a sunscreen, be sure that it has broad-spectrum UV protection (containing UVA and UVB filters).

3.   Avoid sunscreens that incorporate a form of Vitamin A, retinyl palmitate (this would involve 41 percent of all sunscreens). According to preliminary data from the FDA (its full report is expected October 2010) and confirmed by the Environmental Working Group, retinyl palmitate, when applied to skin in the presence of sunlight, acts as a photocarcinogen and hastens the development of skin tumors and lesions. Other forms of Vitamin A, such as retinol, retinyl acetate, and other retinyls, in other sunscreens or cosmetic products should be avoided as they are expected to display common toxic properties. This prohibition does not apply to carotenoids (plant-based compounds that are converted to Vitamin A in the body) that are not toxic when ingested with plant foods or when applied on the skin.

4.   As discussed in chapter 8, many skin creams and ointments have toxins that may be a contributing factor in the development of cancer and other diseases; sunscreens are no different. Most contain toxic chemicals that cause allergic reactions and are hormone disrupters. There are mineral and non-mineral formulations of sunscreens. Although there is no ingredient in sunscreens that is without hazard, after a review of the scientific literature, EWG favored the use of mineral sunscreens (containing zinc oxide or titanium dioxide) because of their low capacity to penetrate the skin and the superior UVA protection they offer. They raised concerns about oxybenzone, the most common active ingredient in sunscreen, found in 60 percent of the 500 beach and sport sunscreens in their 2010 database, because of its ability to penetrate the skin and its association with allergic reactions and potential hormone disruption. This chemical has been detected in 96 percent of the U.S. population (see Table 9.3).

What You Can't See Might Hurt You

In the emergency room, I've seen many parents bring small children to be evaluated after they have fallen and struck their head, or they are experiencing acute abdominal pain. Sometimes, these parents have insisted that a CT (computed tomography) scan be done, in the belief that such an exam is benign and would lead to a more accurate and thorough diagnosis. I have also read advertisements claiming that whole-body CT scans are a valuable component in a total wellness exam because they may provide early detection of a disease. But exposing everyone to increasing amounts of such radiation can have damaging effects, particularly as we age.

My colleague Dr. David West, from Bellevue Hospital, was gracious enough to write about the risks from these ionizing radiation exposures for this book. As an experienced radiologist, he offers a valuable perspective about the issue. His remarks: "advancing to the forefront in media reports is the health risk from exposure to ionizing radiation. We are exposed to ionizing radiation from a variety of procedures including X-rays, CT (computed tomography) scans, angiography (such as cardiac stents), mammography, and fluoroscopy (real time x-rays). There has been an explosion in medical imaging in the United States. In fact, 70 million CT scans are performed every year. This is a 2300% increase in CT scans since 1980.

No prospective scientific studies (the gold standard of modern medicine) have been performed to evaluate the risks, due to ethical concerns about exposing patients to something believed to be harmful. The risks of radiation exposure are therefore extrapolated from data obtained from atomic-bomb survivors in Japan.

It is estimated that 29,000 people in the United States will get cancer as a result of their CT scans every year. That is a staggering number of people, each representing someone's mother, father, child, or friend.

Ionizing radiation causes damage to DNA; the particles of energy cause the strands of DNA to break apart. While our bodies have mechanisms to repair the damage, not all of it can be corrected. Some of the damaged cells will eventually turn cancerous and grow uncontrolled.

Not all radiation is necessarily bad. Some scientists theorize, using hysteresis theory (a memory or lagging effect), that a certain amount of radiation is beneficial because it ramps up our DNA repair systems. We are all exposed to ionizing radiation from nature; specifically, we each average 2.4 millirem of background exposure each year.

Traveling from coast to coast in an airplane can expose us to an additional one to two millirem per flight. However, the radiation exposure from medical procedures varies tremendously, from a low of 10 mrem for a simple chest x-ray to 1000 mrem for a CT scan of the pelvis to up to 5700 mrem for angioplasty.

The dramatic increase in the number of CT scans in the United States has come about for a number of reasons.

In American culture, physicians are held by many patients to the unrealistic expectation of perfection. In fact, I had one patient, who threatened a lawsuit for a perceived medical error, tell me to my face, "I pay you to be perfect." You must remember that all physicians are human and none of us are perfect. In addition, some physicians are also investors in imaging equipment and they engage in self-referral, which is a dirty little secret of the medical community. These physicians can make as much or more money from self-referral of imaging than they make in the actual practice of medicine.

What can you do to mitigate your exposure to potentially harmful medical procedures? First, consider alternative imaging techniques. Magnetic resonance imaging (MRI) uses powerful magnets rather than ionizing radiation to obtain exquisitely detailed images. Ultrasound uses sound waves. Neither of these two modalities causes the DNA damage that ionizing radiation does.

Second, consider if the test is truly medically necessary. If it is, the benefits will far outweigh the risk of radiation. To address the concern about unneeded medical tests, The American College of Radiology has developed a very extensive system of appropriateness criteria. If this system were followed by all doctors, we would be exposed to far less radiation. Be sure to ask if the institution follows these well-established criteria.

Third, The American College of Radiology was chosen by Medicare to oversee accreditation for all types of medical imaging. Accreditation involves a rigorous review of nationally accepted standards to ensure that, not only do the equipment and images meet peer approval, but the interpreting physician is qualified and certified. Be sure to ask if the institution where you are receiving your scan takes the time and effort to be peer reviewed and approved. Or do they just do as they please? There is no monetary reward for accreditation, only the satisfaction, as a physician and as an institution, that the standards followed have been reviewed and approved by an impartial third party.

You can also ask if the institution is being proactive regarding your radiation exposure. Does the staff track your cumulative radiation exposure, providing you or your doctor with warnings over a certain level? Do they have procedures in place to monitor protocols to avoid radiation over-dosage arising from technical errors (this recently happened at Cedars Sinai Medical Center in Los Angeles, which by any physician's estimation is a premier institute). Institutions do not get paid extra to monitor your radiation exposure; if they do have these procedures in place, it indicates they have your interests at heart, at least on this one issue.

It is your body and you have the right to make any and all decisions regarding it. The next time a test is ordered that involves ionizing radiation, ask your doctor if it is necessary, what new or additional information is to be obtained, and if there are any reasonable alternatives.

However, just as receiving unwarranted medical tests can be harmful, your refusal of a truly necessary medical test can be even more harmful. Always remember, if a medical test involving radiation is medically warranted, the benefit far outweighs the risk."

Your Biology is Your Biography

I cannot overemphasize the importance of attitude in resolving chronic health conditions. It starts with accepting responsibility for your health. Only you have the power to implement changes that will improve an ongoing health problem. You deserve to enjoy an exuberant and flourishing state of physical wholeness.

The choices you made up until now have brought you to your current state of health. The choices you make, starting today, will either continue this trend or improve it. It's all up to you.

Another masterful attitude comes from believing that you truly can triumph over a chronic condition to achieve even greater health. These two attitudes, combined together, will drive you toward choices that bring about exactly what you believe. It is always this way. Read the section on epigenetics in chapters 7 and 8 if you need more convincing.

If you are truly committed to aging to perfection, then you need to actively guard your health in all ways. Uncontrolled conditions simply don't fit into this picture. High blood pressure and diabetes are two examples; left unaddressed, they will shorten your lifespan. These are examples of circumstances directly under your control. The former is resolvable with healthy living practices; the latter, sometimes a lifetime challenge, responds to changes only you can make.

There are many conditions leading to high blood pressure and they all come down to stress. Obesity and an unhealthy diet, lack of exercise, and unremitting daily pressure from work or family issues are the kinds of stressors that cause high blood pressure. Read chapter 5 for an understanding of how chronic stress is a killer.

If your stressors are always on, then you will gain weight because cortisol increases blood sugar. You will start to pack it on, especially in the belly, and excess weight starts an unhealthy spiral into high blood pressure. Manage the stress and the weight. They are connected at the hip.

You must also control your LDL cholesterol, which builds up in your arteries and narrows them. High blood pressure, or hypertension, may initially cause no symptoms but will slowly destroy your quality of life. The effect of hypertension is not just restricted to one organ; it leads to blood-vessel damage everywhere from the pounding going on throughout the arteries in your body. In the kidneys, you start leaking proteins and blood; your renal indices go up, indicating damage; and your kidneys fail. The same is true for your liver. In your brain, the increased pressure leads eventually to a stroke and irreversible damage.

I like to bridge the two worlds of traditional medicine and alternative or complementary medicine. It is a type of "east meets west" approach. There is a place for both. If someone comes in with high blood pressure, this is going to kill him first and I need to get it under control with medication. I will prescribe traditional medicines when needed because otherwise he may die of a heart attack tomorrow, before I ever get the chance to balance his hormones and improve his lifestyle issues. Sometime down the road I will slowly wean him off that medication completely. And he will come off those pills, if he truly desires to be healthy.

High blood pressure combined with an existing diabetes condition leads to an exponential increase in the damage that occurs. Unfortunately, these two conditions are almost always in combination. If you have diabetes, you will develop high blood pressure; if you have high blood pressure, you may very well develop diabetes from damage to the pancreas and the impaired ability to make insulin.

Bioidentical Support for Diabetes

Dan Pang's diabetes, complicated by obesity, wreaked havoc in his life and there didn't seem to be anything he could do about it. A severe diabetic, he faced a life sentence of pain and ill health but bioidentical hormone therapy helped to turn this around. This is his story.

Diabetes-related pain in his legs was so excruciating that Dan was taking some very powerful drugs to manage it. "I had put on a lot of weight as a result of not being able to exercise properly. I tried numerous ways to lose the weight and get myself back into a more healthy condition but nothing I tried seemed to work," he says. Frustration at this failure and the ongoing pain drove Dan deeper into a black depression.

After a full assessment, I recommended bioidentical testosterone therapy. "Within days I started to notice that my thought process became very acute and focused," he says. Dan's mood steadily improved, his depression began fading, and his physical well-being soared. "With a drive inside me that I hadn't felt in years, I started an exercise program in my living room. My need for insulin started to drastically drop and so did the extra weight."

His physical stamina slowly improved and daily walks became his new lifestyle. "The pain that I had been experiencing faded from my legs and I was able to remove the powerful medications from my life." Dan worked very hard to turn his health around, but now his bioidentical hormones were supporting his efforts. "In my first six months with Dr. Garcia I was able to lose 40 pounds and now am able to run a mile three days a week."

The most rewarding benefit of his new health is being able to "run and play in the park with my seven year old son. Nobody has to convince me that the program works. I've seen unbelievable results in my life," Dan says.

Habitual Addictions

When you drink a lot of caffeine or eat a high-carbohydrate, sugar-laden snack, you are trying to increase your levels of the neurotransmitter serotonin. When you eat for comfort because you have no friends or are lonely, you are also trying to increase serotonin to make you feel better. This hormone has a calming or anxiety-reducing effect. At my addiction clinic, I've seen the results in heroin addicts who are trying to do the same thing: increase the release of neurotransmitters by ingesting a substance.

There is a certain temporary pleasure in such a habit, but it's misread by the body. Whether it's an addiction to smoking, food, sex, or heroin, it all comes down to the same thing: an effort to increase the neurotransmitters in your brain. But these health-robbing habits increase the stress in your body, leading to its breakdown over a period of time.

People who succeed in giving up such a habit might have watched a show, or had a family member help them, or they just became tired of feeling sick and tired. You have to make the decision to change your life. Sometimes that means getting help from a coach like me, or from family or friends, or through joining an addiction program.

A patient who was anorexic early in her life got over it because of the love and help from a family who nurtured her, comforted her, and insisted that she do some things she didn't want to do. She's now fine, but without this help she could have died. She was very grateful for the intervention.

It's like dieting with a co-worker. The chances of success are going to be much greater because someone is encouraging you. I've seen people who have just stopped smoking cold turkey, but that's the exception. I think it's much easier and your chances of success are greater if you do it with help from people around you.

Helping the Healing

Why are some people who have everything in the world depressed? And why is it that some people who have nothing are simply happy? It's how you perceive things and the attitude you bring to your life: being grateful for what you have. I think it all starts in the brain and then the body follows.

My father grew up on the border between Guatemala and Mexico in a family of twelve with absolutely nothing. Their bathtub was a nearby stream and Abe Lincoln's log cabin would be a palace compared to his house. You can imagine its primitive nature but he tells me that it was the best time of his life.

At six months of age, we immigrated to Texas. They came to the United States without knowing a word of English. They started from nothing and have lived the American dream. Through their sacrifices, they raised four children who became very successful.

Some people who were born in this wonderful country, with all its advantages, having always lived a life of privilege, have absolutely no motivation to do anything. I think sometimes you need a little challenge; you need failure and success to appreciate where you've been and where you've gone. When it has all been simply given to you, you tend to lose your motivation.

I spent two years in Kindergarten learning how to speak English. That kind of challenge, followed by success, is very motivating. The challenge of improving your health, if you approach it with the right mind, can generate the same kind of enthusiasm.

My father has maintained that "merry heart" I described in chapter 7; he has a simple appreciation and wonder of the world that makes him enjoy life as much as he can. I inherited a lot of that attitude from my parents and it made me profoundly open to experiencing whatever life had to teach me.

From the time I could walk, I remember my grandfather taking me to the open markets commonly found in most Mexican villages. We bought natural, organic food daily for our meals. I enjoyed the intimate, direct experience of buying food from those who grew it. I gained an appreciation of simple, wholesome foods and exposure to a more natural lifestyle. It made me open to alternatives.

I have combined the best of both cultures (my heritage and medical training) in my approach to healing: the new world and the old world; the allopathic, traditional medicine of my hospital training and the more intimate, osteopathic, and holistic philosophies of alternative and functional medicine. I have straddled both approaches ever since. It can be a challenge, but my background made me want to combine all that I have learned in pursuit of healing.

In the tradition of massage, reflexology, and chiropractic, as an osteopathic physician, I always touch my patients. I learned that the sterile, antiseptic quality of a hospital setting can actually inhibit healing; it can keep loved ones away from the patient and create fear. So I take the time to connect with my patients, quell their anxiety, and encourage them.

As Beverly Lauder recalls, her treatment for hot flashes, skin and vaginal dryness, loss of libido, fatigue, and insomnia began as a long chat with me. "It was a talking appointment. I did a lot of talking," she says with a smile. She recalls me doing a lot of listening and taking notes.

"From what I told him and from the lab tests, Dr. Garcia suggested some vitamins, minerals, most of it over-the-counter, and prescriptions for very small, safe doses of oral and topical bioidentical hormone creams to be taken or applied once a day. We talked about exercise and its importance, even just regular walking. He explained the results of the tests and what they meant. And he told me that my complaints could be fixed."

Even at the age of 67, Beverly remembers that there was nothing I suggested that she could not do. She remembers hearing everything I said. "But I especially heard that we, together, could relieve these symptoms." My willingness to help her, to spend some time talking to her and support her in working through a maze of intimidating health challenges, was tremendously encouraging for Beverly.

In modern, Western medicine, we have lost our way. We are humans, not machines, and medical science is no substitute for the human touch. I'm a physician first, looking for every possible way to heal my patient. You can heal people by talking to them in a compassionate way, and knowing that someone cares about them. These types of small steps make huge differences in a person's life. You will never know how much you affected another person just by encouraging them.

Table 9.3:

Sunscreens with highest concern for human exposure and toxicity

Sunscreen chemical
Percent of U.S. sunscreens containing it
Exposure (skin penetration and biomonitoring)
Toxicity concerns

4-Methylbenzylidene camphor (4-MBC)	FDA approval pending. Limited skin penetration (1%) *in vivo.* Detected in European mothers' milk at low parts per billion levels. Strong evidence of hormone disruption; thyroid effects;[5] behavioral alterations in female rats.
Benzophenone-3 (oxybenzone)	60%. 1-9% absorbed according to *in vivo* skin studies; detected in volunteers' urine and in European mothers' milk. Present in 96% of Americans' urine; higher maternal exposures are associated with a decrease in birth weight for girls and an increase in boys. Hormone disruption; reproductive effects and altered organ weights in chronic feeding studies. High rates of photo-allergy.
3-Benzylidene camphor	FDA approval pending. Hormone disruption; *in vivo* effects—behavior and estrous cycling.

Octyl methoxycinnamate (OMC)	40%. Limited skin penetration *in vivo* <1%, urine, and in European mothers' milk at low parts per billion levels.[4] Multiple estrogenic effects. Thyroid hormone reductions; and hormone-mediated immune effects. Moderate rates of skin allergy. {Rodriguez, 2006 #2683}
Padimate O	1.0%. Limited skin penetration. Detected in European mothers' milk at low parts per billion levels. Estrogenic effects. Damages DNA; causes allergic reactions in some people.

Sunscreens with moderate concern for human exposure and toxicity

Octocrylene	49%. Limited skin penetration in vivo. Detected in European mothers' milk. Slight to moderate skin irritation.
Ensulizole	1.2%. Skin penetration measured in vivo, documented concentrations in urine. Occasional photoallergic reactions reported.
Homosalate	45% Limited skin penetration in vivo <1% Not detected in European mothers' milk. Limited evidence of hormone disruption. Toxic metabolites.
Sulisobenzone (Benzophenone-4)	0.2% Skin penetration measured, estimated at 1% Limited evidence of hormone disruption.
Zinc Oxide	29%. Very limited skin penetration. Estimated at 0.4% in volunteers for nano - and conventional particle sizes. Unknown whether it is in elementa

(harmless) or insoluble particle form (toxicologically harmful). No photoallergy or hormone disruption. Skin cell study found zinc nanoparticles provoked oxidative stress and DNA damage. Coatings may reduce skin reactivity. Zinc inhalation causes lung inflammation.

Titanium Dioxide	28%. Very limited skin penetration; penetration of hairless mouse skin; no skin penetration in min-pigs. No photoallergy or hormone disruption. Probable carcinogen when inhaled. Inhaled nanoparticles reach organs, cross placenta, and enter brain. Skin damage in vitro.[48]

Sunscreens with lowest concern for human exposure and toxicity

Avobenzone	50%. Limited skin penetration *in vivo;* and *in vitro (0.8%)*. No evidence of photoallergy or hormone disruption.
Mexoryl SX	Limited approval (4 formulations); broader FDA approval pending. Limited skin penetration *in vivo (0.16%)*. No evidence of hormone disruption. Rarely reported skin allergy, more often in children.
Octisalate	59%. Limited skin penetration *in vivo* <1% and *in vitro* (~0.5%) Rarely, allergic contact dermatitis.
Tinosorb M	FDA approval pending. Low skin penetration measured *in vitro*. No *in vitro* hormone effects. Did not stimulate uterotrophic activity in vivo. Allergic reactions uncommon.

| Tinosorb S | FDA approval pending. No *in vitro* hormone effects; did not stimulate uterotrophic activity. |

• Four other ingredients approved in the United States are almost never used in sunscreen, and are poorly studied: Menthyl Anthranilate, Benzophenone-8, PABA, and Trolamine salicylate.

Taken from Environmental Working Group. *EWG's 2010 Sunscreen Guide.*

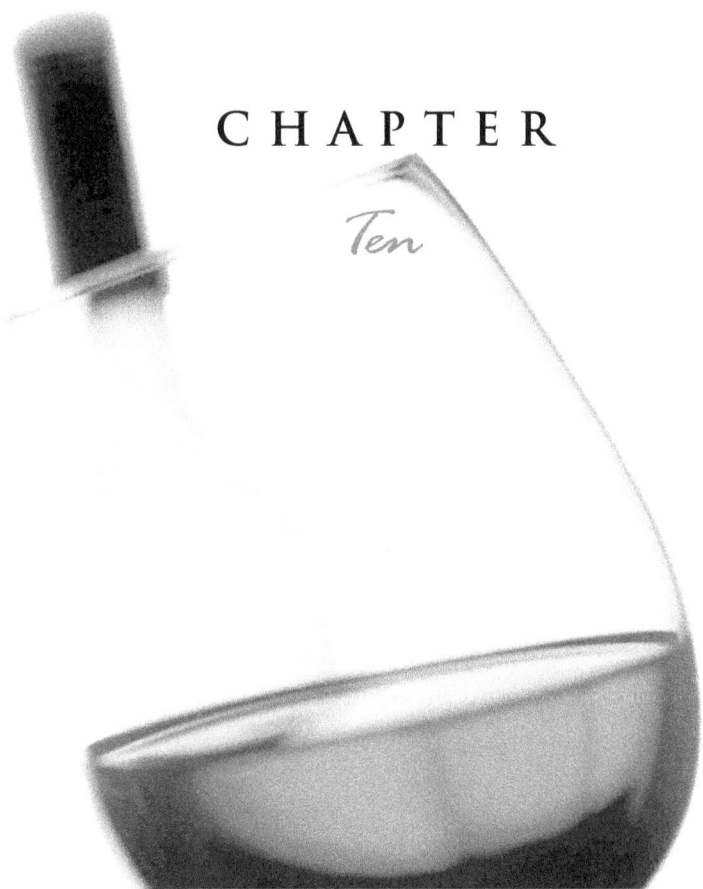

CHAPTER

Ten

CHAPTER 10

Master Your Maturity

*"At seventy you are but a child, at eighty you are merely
a youth, and at ninety if the ancestors invite you into
heaven, ask them to wait until you are one hundred
and then you might consider it."*

*Proverb carved into stone marker
on an Okinawa beach*

The purpose of this book has been to show you that it's okay to age.
You don't have to be 20 years old forever, doing all those things
necessary to appear young. If you want to, that's fine. But you can
still celebrate your age.

Life is all about change. You've reached a point where you are comfortable in
so many ways; so honor where you're at right now, instead of where you've
been. Age to perfection. Don't read *Glamour* magazine and believe that you

must look like that when you're 50. It's not going to happen! But having a fit and healthy body, at an appropriate weight, with dynamic mobility, freedom from age-related diseases, a clear, sharp intellect, and plenty of energy and enthusiasm for life: these are all realistic.

Life is an evolution that we all go through, and it's exciting at every stage. The key is protecting your strength and valuable health so that you can enjoy all the days to come.

Some people say that we have turned menopause into a disease for the purpose of creating a market for bioidentical hormones. In fact, some have asked, "Why are we doing this when people have always lived with this condition?" Such thinking is a little misguided because you could say the same about many other conditions. For example, "People have been dying of heart attacks forever, so why are we saving them now, and why are we giving them anti-hypertensive medication, bypasses and angioplasty? Just let them die." Both of these are age-related discomforts.

Hormones are intimately connected to who we are. They comprise our metabolic rate, our sexual identity, our ability to perceive the world and stressors affecting us, and our ability to reproduce. Anything affecting the body's health will affect our hormones however, the challenges we face in middle age today, were mostly unknown a century ago. Our ancestors didn't suffer in the same way because most didn't live long enough to experience how declining hormonal levels can destroy health. The increasing toxicity of our environment, combined with stressful lifestyles and sedentary jobs, all help to inhibit aging to perfection.

I only need to look at my many confused and worried, older patients to know that it is a quality-of-life issue. Keeping our longer-lived bodies vigorously strong and healthy requires a life-supporting program of bioidentical hormone therapy, ample exercise, optimal nutrition, stress reduction, and a very positive, productive attitude.

Manage your maturity with this combination; it can change your whole outlook. Once you have that joy in your life, you will feel like you can accomplish anything. They say that, in anyone's life, we will have seven different careers. I've done that already, and I am in my mid-fifties. I've been through seven careers and have found that it's constantly exciting; the possibilities are endless. It's like falling in love: everything feels great, and you get up in the morning energized and looking forward to each day. The same can be true of new relationships or any other challenge, as long as you're fit, healthy, and vitally alive.

You want to maintain a youthful appearance, confident demeanor, and an attitude that you can accomplish anything; the goal is to be active, vibrant, and alive through your nineties, and then continue on into another century of living. In 10 or 15 years, reports indicate that people will routinely live to between 110 and 150 because of breakthroughs in advanced nutraceuticals, stem cell applications, bioengineering, and nanotechnology. Who wants to live those last 50 years in a nursing home? Not you; you want to be vibrantly alive, discovering new aspects of your world, and thoroughly enjoying yourself.

Renowned inventor and futurist Ray Kurzweil co-authored *Fantastic Voyage: Live Long Enough to Live Forever* with Terry Grossman. Its basic premise is that, if middle-aged people can live long enough, degenerative diseases and even old age will soon be overcome. If you plot the pace of innovation and knowledge along a curve, it becomes clear that larger time periods in history produced relatively small advances in knowledge. But within the steeper portion of that curve, the place where we currently are, astronomical developments are happening within increasingly short periods of time.

Our rate of growth is not linear anymore; it's exponential. We are doubling our knowledge every year or so, a pace of advancement that used to take three centuries. For example, "It took fourteen years to sequence the HIV virus, but we sequenced the SARS virus in thirty-one days," Kurzweil says. We literally cannot predict what will occur over the next 10 or 15 years. It will be that radical a change.

We now have artificial joints to replace ones that wear out. As adults, we have stem cells within our bones; research into these cells offers the promise of regenerating our immune system and organs such as the heart and kidneys. If they fail, we could grow another one. Scientists are using our own intrinsic ability to regenerate ourselves. From stem-cell research to advances in energy medicine, we're redefining the expression of our genes in ways never thought possible.

Your family history and your genetic makeup are only 25 percent of your risk factors for aging. You have 75 percent control over the quality of your future health and vitality. Three-quarters of your healthful future depend on your ability to change or redirect your life the way you want to. Through this book, I've been supplying a lot of the education you need to do this, but you must supply the motivation. Maybe you just have to get to a point where you feel so bad that you finally want to know what it was like when you were 20 years old again...when you felt great.

You can overcome everything in your physiology through your psychology: what you think influences the choices you make. Your attitude is critically important to how you perceive the opportunities in your world.

If you want to change your life, let go of the bad things that happened to you. We're all affected by things that happened in our lives, including myself. You must stop punishing yourself or thinking about the past. Somehow, you just have to find a way to let it go and get back to who you were. I'm able to do it, in part because of the hormones I'm on, but also because of my attitude.

Doing it requires an across-the-board combination of actions: from exercising to new relationships to stress-reducing practices such as yoga, meditation, religion, or creative visualization. You can release the trauma so that the person you once knew can come out again. Future innovations in the field of energy medicine offer the promise of releasing trauma in seconds by working with the body's energy waves, down to the cellular level. Wow.

Time to Change

Right now, you want to immediately halt the aging process and enjoy a superb state of vitality and stamina. Most people don't want to wait years to see results, and they won't have to, but we live in a society that wants a quick, one-pill fix and immediate results. It's just not that way when it comes to health; it takes a little time.

I'm not talking years, but mere months, before you start feeling and looking better. This is about a permanent life fix that will last for the rest of your days. I don't have a fountain of youth pill to offer you; just a fountain of youth lifestyle. As with weight loss, you want to change slowly so that lasts. You want to feel better for the rest of your life. The changes I've discussed do work, but how fast it will happen depends on how badly you have treated your body.

Men often respond much more quickly than women, but the impatience is the same. Greg Davis was typical of the North American desire for rapid results. At the age of 49, Greg was wondering if his best years were over. "I was struggling for the energy to make it through three workouts a week at the gym and my job as an on-call charter jet pilot was wearing me down," he recalls. Having lived a healthy lifestyle with rigorous strength training at its core, he was losing muscle tone and suffered from chronic joint and back pain as well as a loss of libido.

"I found it disheartening to watch myself slowly backslide through my forties instead of making gains or at least maintaining the level I had already achieved. I couldn't help but wonder how much more my physical activities would fade as I entered my fifties," he says. When Greg heard about bioidentical hormone replacement, "It was as if a light bulb went off in my head." He did some research online and became so motivated that he willingly drove three hours to be treated by me. "I thought if this really works, well, a three-hour drive is not that big a sacrifice."

We reviewed his health history and I created a program suited to his needs involving bioidentical testosterone cream and nutraceuticals. But Greg was very impatient to see results. "The day I received my supplements, I drove to the gym thinking that I'd be an instant iron man again! Well, it didn't quite work that way. I must admit that I was a tad disappointed." I had warned Greg to give it a few weeks, and he started listening. Then the results began arriving.

"Gradually, without really noticing at first, my workouts at the gym improved. An hour and a half seemed to fly by and I had to tell myself to go home as there was still energy left in me. I was actually adding weight to the bar instead of taking it off." He was delighted at the return of his muscle definition, strength, and stamina. "It was as if years were lifted away. The aches and pains in my joints were also lessened. I am rolling into age 51 this year like a freight train. And to think just rubbing on a cream and swallowing some supplements could do that. It's sweet!"

"Oh, and one other benefit is that my libido has returned to that of a thirty-year-old again. Nice perk, eh?" Greg says he's "starting to get used to people guessing my age as early forties." He comes for checkups several times a year. "Dr. Garcia is constantly monitoring and fine tuning to keep me at optimum levels of health. You don't find many physicians like him," he says. Greg encourages others to get on the bioidentical health train, adding, "Everyone deserves to feel their best!"

Women, with their more complex hormonal chemistry, may take six months to a year to completely rebalance their hormones. I always have to reduce their expectation of quick results. They always think that within a week they'll be like a completely new woman. It doesn't happen that way. Their body has taken a long time to get so sick and it takes some time to get back their health.

I always recheck them in three months and ask, "Give me a percentage of how much you've improved." A report of zero is rare; usually the rate of improvement at this point is 30 to 50 percent. Then I encourage them by saying, "Listen, this is just the beginning."

Your body has a remarkable ability to make up for what you are not giving it. But at some point you start getting sick. The same thing is true on the way back. You're so depleted of hormones, nutrients, and energy that the foundation needs to be rebuilt. It's like trying to lose weight. You don't lose 10 pounds in the first week; you lose 10 pounds in the first month.

I have seen it happen over and over again. It takes some time and then something happens: the switches get turned on. Lights start coming on in a room you've never had before. Before you know it, your whole house is lit up again.

I think the people who appreciate the change most are the family and friends who notice a change in a patient's activity level; he or she becomes more interested, focused, and engaged with life. They start reaching out more to their relatives, friends, and their community and that's positively reinforcing, allowing them to come out of their doldrums. The contrast between this and a previously withdrawn person can be dramatic.

For Lindsay Anders, isolation caused by hormonal imbalance eventually wrecked her marriage. The 52-year-old was suffering from progesterone deficiency so severe that her levels of this hormone were bottomed out. "I began to feel lonely and disconnected from my husband, children, family, and friends, not wanting to be around anyone. It was so difficult to feel cut off from the world and yet there seemed like no obvious reason that this was happening," Lindsay recalls.

Her 32-year-old marriage began to crumble. "It became so pronounced that I left home twice, briefly, renting my own apartment so I could be alone to figure out what was going on with my mind." I treated her with bioidentical progesterone cream and adrenal supplements. I urged her to adopt a program of good nutrition and exercise, and to be patient.

Then it happened. "Wow! Within three months, I was my previous self again, enjoying people, my profession, and living each day to the fullest with gratitude to my God each morning as I awoke from a good night's sleep," she says. Although her marriage ended, Lindsay found a new direction for her world. With renewed energy levels she led an increasingly upbeat lifestyle. "It allowed me to become active in the gym, training clients as a personal trainer," she says.

Emotional or physical isolation, like the kind Lindsay experienced, is tremendously aging. Lack of energy and not feeling well can sap your desire to connect with others. It can creep up on you slowly. When you are self-focused and not oriented to your community, it is very easy to get into a depressive rut. It sends messages to your brain to start expressing the genes for depression, and there are 250 genes influenced by depression alone.

But when you are feeling healthy and exuberant, with the "happy heart" that I've talked about, it fires off different genes that continue to enhance your wellness. Everything just works better. You have a sense of peace, a connection to the world, and a satisfaction with your community.

In *The Blue Zones*, by Dan Buettner, the centenarians profiled from the Okinawans in Japan to the Sardinians in Italy to the Nicoyans of Costa Rica and the Seventh Day Adventists in Southern California, all place a high emphasis on family and friends. They look forward to family gatherings and get together regularly with friends, often daily, to share a laugh and talk about their community. Each has a culture that values a healthy diet and exercise but also being of service to others.

If you live a self-centered life, you won't expand your horizons to include the possibilities other people can bring into your world. Your health and longevity both benefit from social interaction. You can start first with family; open up communication with your children, parents, or partner, and it can unlock other miracles in your life.

The "blue zone" communities highlight how feelings of self-worth are fed by having satisfying relationships with family and community. Get started by joining a ski club, walking club, or any other kind of club that enables you to meet people. Interaction is uplifting; it lifts depression and makes you feel like you are part of something bigger than yourself.

We are all trying to find our place in the world. Why not make it an adventure, or something stimulating that invigorates you? You can be as exciting at 80 as you were at 20. You just have to make a little effort and expand your horizons. Then you have the benefit of growing your mind and increasing those important synapses between neurocells with new things and new people. That is anti-aging in itself. That is your own "blue zone."

Your mind will never go into dementia or depression; you will remain alert and enthusiastic about life. There are a lot of similarities between the addicted brain and the isolated brain. In both cases, brain hormones such as serotonin and dopamine drop; focus gets impaired and pleasure receptors decline. It proves that we all need social interaction to age with youthful health and vitality.

They Inspire Us

People who are aged to perfection, enjoy a strong, fit body that is not overweight; they move with ease, and they converse with alert poise. They are good conversationalists, engaging and robustly alive, and a source of inspiration to others. They think of themselves as much younger; at 70 they feel like they are 30 or 40.

You want to be near them, and invite them over. You want to know more about them and are always learning from them. They are so interesting that you can talk to them forever and you just want to be like them.

Someone said to me the other day, "Roger, I feared being in my fifties until I met you, because I thought it would mean slowing down, not being able to move well, and no longer being able to live out my dreams. But you act much younger than a man in his fifties." I still think that I'm 30.

For many people, their conception of age is being old and decrepit, fading away in a nursing home, all alone. That is not my conception of age at all. Mine is about remaining vigorously strong and active, socially and sexually, and thinking young.

I've found that helping people to change their whole aging process is tremendously rewarding. I keep hearing the same thing: "Doctor, I've finally found the person I used to be." Their world is not so dull and grey any more. It's like color television over the black-and-white sets we used to have. In my emergency-room work, it's rare to feel that I've made the same kind of difference in people's lives.

Tips to Add Years to Your Life

Eat less. Fewer calories are shown to increase life expectancy. Eat more vegetables; they are loaded with protective antioxidants. Eat fresh, not processed, foods; they are higher in nutrients, while packaged foods tend to contain a lot of additives.

Exercise regularly. It enhances all metabolic, hormonal, mental, and immune processes.

Practice optimism. A positive outlook in life is associated with longevity and influences how well you will age. Denial and fear of aging will accelerate the degenerative process. Practice a positive attitude about growing older; a recent study shows this could add an average of 7.5 years to your life. *Ragtime* composer Eubie Blake, when he hit 100, joked, "If I had known I was going to live this long, I would have taken better care of myself." You're never too young to think about healthy aging. Your risk for an unhealthy future can be greatly lowered through lifestyle choices you start making today.

Forget about a "what's the use" mindset. No matter how long you have been a junk-food junkie or couch potato, it is never too late to enhance your quality of life. Family history and genetics count for about 25 percent of your life expectancy; you control the other 75 percent with a combination of nutrition, physical activity, and attitude.

Nurture your spirit. Studies on centenarians all over the world have found that spirituality and a sense of humor are the most common traits of people who live past the age of 100, no matter their social circumstances.

Recognize that you're not alone; we are in a tsunami-wave of aging. Every eight seconds, someone in the United States turns 50. Embrace your membership in this growing club; take pride in your ability to choose a healthy, active lifestyle that supports your maturity.

Read books. Learn a lot of new things. Stimulating the mind helps to keep it sharp. Enjoy being creative and appreciating the creativity of others; art and music enhance brain functioning.

Get married. People who are married tend to live longer than those who are single.

Watch your weight. Excess weight and the insulin resistance it brings increase the risk of diabetes, heart disease, and cancer, all diseases that reduce longevity.

Moderation is Marvelous

It's not absolutely necessary to stay on a plant-based diet for the rest of your life. Moderation is the key, as in all things. You can have some meat if you eat organically; you can have a little bit of all the foods that make life pleasurable. Don't be a monk about this stuff. You have to live in the 21st century.

No one says that you can't have cake on your birthday. If you restrict yourself by living a completely pure lifestyle that includes every single point I've made, you likely wouldn't enjoy yourself at all. It's all about living in moderation, maybe six days a week. Eat cheeseburgers in moderation. I do, although I try to make them organic beef. Of course, that's hard to do during long shifts in the emergency department. It's all a balancing act, for me and for you.

So find your balance and set your intention to be like a seagull. A seagull, from the moment it's born to the moment of death, is always at 100 percent. These birds all just die at 100 percent. That's what I want to be: going along at 100 percent and then boom! I am simply dead, having lived to the age of 130. Now that's aging to perfection.

Afterword

The journey through the many topics I have outlined in the book very likely is a new one for many of you. The concepts are very different from those you may have read about or discussed with your doctor and certainly different from those I was taught in medical school. It is an acknowledgment that the confines of traditional allopathic medicine has not been altogether successful in keeping us healthy. Despite all the advantages of new technology, research, new medicines and state-of-the-art diagnostic lab and equipment, we as a population are getting sicker and sicker. We are living longer but the quality of that life is increasingly compromised by pain, immobility, dementia, depression, diminished eyesight and hearing. The human costs and financial resources that will be needed to care for the coming aging of America with these conditions will be staggering. (The Census Bureau projects that the number of Americans age 65 or older will double in the next 25 years, representing 20% of the total population with people age 85 or older, the fastest growing segment of the population.)

Seeking answers not found within conventional medicine, many people have turned to unconventional therapies. These new modalities of healing have been globally described as complementary and alternative medicine (CAM). As a testament to their desire to find something that works, 38% of adults and 12% of children in the United States are using some form of CAM as revealed by the 2007 National Health Interview Survey (NHIS). Why is CAM popular? Perhaps it is the time that these practitioners spend with their patients, that they touch their patients and that there is a recognition that true wellness is achieved only by bringing forth the power of the interaction between the body, mind and spirit.

This new paradigm shift is also occurring within conventional medicine today. People are demanding more than the usual "one size fits all" approach. Knee-jerk reactions to the treatment of symptoms of illness in of itself is no longer adequate. Integrative and functional medicine physicians understand this as their focus is on wellness and not sickness. This wellness concept describes health as the optimal functioning of all organ systems with prevention a priority rather than simply looking at health as the absence of disease. When illness does arrive, sorting out its root cause is paramount, not just treatment that masks the symptoms.

This paradigm shift also involves a two-way conversation with patients. You must take responsibility for your health by making good lifestyle choices. We know that a lifetime of poor personal choices, poor diet, lack of exercise and stress is a proven recipe for chronic disease, disability and a premature death. You must choose good habits, not bad ones. Our environment has been degraded enough without compounding our toxicity through our own hand. Make a habit of exercise, eating organically, getting good sleep, fostering optimism and nurturing your spiritual side. Eliminate the habits of drug and alcohol use, smoking, eating processed and GMO food, a stressful lifestyle where there is no room for exercise, staying up late and pessimism.

I wrote Aged to Perfection to serve as a roadmap for your journey to optimal health and vitality. That despite our compromised food, air and water quality and the stresses found in the 21st century, it is still possible to age well but it does take some planning and motivation. Just apply the same step-by-step approach you took to fund your retirement but apply it also to your "health fund" on a daily basis. It requires a daily commitment to make time for health. My goal has been to show you this path but only you can take the necessary steps to follow it. By doing so, you will reap the rewards of a great quality of life as you age backwards. There is no need to fear the horizon—you should embrace it! Good aging is not a contraction but an expansion to your life. You can take your hard-won wisdom and experience as well as retain all the things you had in your youth… your memory, vitality, sexuality, mobility and strength, well into your centennial years. You will then experience the joy of youthful aging and not "grow old".

Together in health,

Roger Garcia

To get in touch with Dr. Garcia, please contact BodyLogicMD of Columbus, 1-877-501- 4**ATP** (4287) or email him at DrGarcia@agedtoperfectionbook.com. You may register for his free newsletter at Agedtoperfectionbook.com. In addition, please see Agedtoperfectionbook. com for information concerning Dr. Garcia's upcoming anti-aging lecture series and book publications.

Patient Testimonials

Note: The names of the people whom have provided testimonials for Dr. Roger Garcia have been changed to protect identities and respect their privacy.

I am a severe diabetic and have had chronic health problems including bypass surgery on my heart. I also, as a complication of my diabetes, experienced severe pain in my legs which required powerful drugs to manage. I had put on a lot of weight as a result of not being able to properly exercise. I tried numerous ways to lose the weight and get myself in a healthy condition but nothing that I tried seemed to work. A friend told me of bodylogicmd in Columbus, Ohio. I figured I had nothing to lose. The staff was very friendly and knowledgeable and made my visit very informative and comfortable. They set me up on a program and within days a started to notice that my thought process became very acute. My mood steadily improved and the depression that I had been feeling about my situation faded away. Slowly my physical condition started to improve and, with a drive inside me that I had not felt in years, and I started an exercise program in my living room. My need for insulin started to drop and so did the weight that I had been putting on. I then started to take walks getting longer and longer each day. The pain that I had been experiencing faded and I was able to remove the powerful pain medications from my life. It took a lot of work on my part but in my first six months with Dr. Garcia I was able to lose 40lbs and now am able to run a mile three days a week. Nobody has to try to convince me of anything, this course of treatment works. I can now run and play in the park with my son and for that Dr. Garcia, I say thanks!

-Donna Dartman

My life has been transformed by bodylogicmd my life has been transformed by bodylogicmd of columbus ohio and thanks to my relationship with dr. Roger garcia. I attended a free seminar in December 2007, unsure whether bodylogicmd and bioidentical hormone therapy was for me. I was intrigued by the approach to optimize lab values and eliminate symptoms. At 30-years old, I had struggled with hypothyroidism for over six years, and doctors either never cared enough to help me properly or they lacked the knowledge as to what optimizing thyroid hormone levels involved. After speaking with Dr. Roger at the seminar, I felt hope for the first time that he would be able to help me. At my first appointment, it was confirmed that my thyroid levels were not optimal on my current medication, and I also learned that I had adrenal fatigue. I appreciated Dr. Roger's genuine ne concern for my wellbeing, as well as his honesty when he asked for more time to research my case and consult his colleagues.

Dr. Roger helped me support my adrenals, which is a critical part of treating hypothyroidism. He also switched me to armour thyroid. He has been willing to experiment with different amounts of armour to determine where I feel best.

With bioidentical hormone therapy, I am now happier, calmer, more energetic, warmer, and sleeping better than I have in years. The year before I saw Dr. Roger, I had not had a period for eleven months. I have already had five periods this year and the year isn't over yet. I finally feel like I am moving in the right direction, now in caring, capable hands. I am grateful to my mother who went with me to the free seminar, and gave me the courage to try the columbus, Ohio-based bodylogicmd. She has also become a patient of Dr. Roger and has had her life turned around as well. I cannot say enough about what Dr. Roger garcia and bodylogicmd have done for my family and I. Thank you!

-Ally Summerhill

*D*r. Roger Garcia is an unusually compassionate doctor. He builds relationships with his patients, earning their trust not only with his vast knowledge of the intricacies of the human body, but also with his genuine interest in striving to help them achieve optimal health. He is also very humble and will admit when he needs more time to research an issue a patient is having or to request additional time to consult with his colleagues to learn how they have successfully helped a patient in a similar situation. Dr. Garcia is willing to try new and innovative methods to achieve health, and although he relies on lab work to guide his decisions, he is always most concerned with how his patients feel and resolving their bothersome symptoms. I first came to Dr. Garcia almost two years ago, unsure if he would be able to help me. I attended a free seminar and was impressed by his unique approach to treating patients and spoke with him briefly afterward, because I was only 30 years old at the time, I didn't know if an anti-aging doctor would be a good fit for me. I had battled for years with a thyroid condition, but never felt like I was able to achieve satisfactory care with my previous doctors. Dr. Garcia's preference of using armour thyroid to treat his patients, combined with his focus on achieving optimal, not just normal lab values, was exactly what I was looking for. After switching my medication and optimizing my dose, I felt like a new person as I regained my health. My energy levels increased, I lost weight, my acne improved, and my periods regulated. What Dr. Garcia has done to improve my quality of life is something that I am thankful for on a daily basis and I am grateful for his effort and commitment to his patients.

-Susan Pliner

*D*epression. Chronic fatigue. Heart rhythm irregularities. Insomnia. Loss of appetite. Weight gain, in spite of little appetite! Non-existent libido. At 53-years of age I felt like my life was over. Years of stress combined with the "normal" aging process had wreaked havoc on my body, mind, and soul. Unbeknownst to me, a trip to New York City to visit some dear friends in October 2006 would be the beginning of an incredible turn around for me. The wife of my dear friend was concerned with my mental state, my inability to think clearly, and the obvious fatigue I was experiencing. She had some experience in nutrition and psychology and had recently heard some wonderful stories about bioidentical hormone therapy. She recommended I see Dr. Roger Garcia at bodylogicmd in Columbus, Ohio, about three hours from my home.

In December 2006 I began bioidentical hormone therapy. Within six weeks I began experiencing a major turnaround. I could sleep. My energy levels were up. The depression began to lift and I could think clearly again. I was beginning to feel like myself again. With the increased energy levels I could begin a regular exercise routine again, and actually began building lean muscle mass and losing a very stubborn layer of abdominal fat that had been building for a number of years. I had my life back again! My wife, my children, and my grandchildren were thrilled to see me emerge from my "dark night of the soul." I was alive again.

I am now approaching the two-year mark since beginning hormone replacement therapy. It will be a part of my daily routine and life from now on. The stress levels of my vocation have not diminished, but my capacity and ability to deal with all the demands has greatly increased. I greatly enjoy biking and have ridden almost 1,200 miles this riding season. Morning prayer and meditation, a regular stretching routine, and a good combination of aerobic and weight bearing exercises, focusing on eating the proper foods, and my daily hormone replacement therapy and supplements have all added up to a brand new me! Thank you lord! Thank you Dr. Roger Garcia!

-George MacArthur

My name is Roberta. I am 55 years old and began experiencing the symptoms of menopause shortly after my 50th birthday. Hot flashes; mood swings and anxiety; night sweats; sleeplessness; fatigue; fuzzy thinking; itching; vaginal dryness and the resulting pain during intercourse, and virtually no libido. I had them all! Every symptom of menopause known man. I tried all of the over-the-counter remedies but none worked for me. I didn't want to take synthetic hrt due to the fear of cancer, but my life had become so unmanageable that I felt I had no choice. I went to my gyn and, of course, I was put on estrogen. The hot flashes, night sweats and sleeplessness began to subside in about 3-4 weeks. However, I still had severe anxiety, irritability and no libido. I had lost my zest for life. Five years ago I lost my daughter in a tragic car accident and am raising her young children. The loss of a child is devastating, but adds the full responsibility for 2 beautiful little girls who had just lost their mother, a demanding career and top it off with menopause. There were times when I thought I was losing my mind. My doctor prescribed an antidepressant. Talk about losing your zest for life, it made me lethargic and miserable. I didn't want to go anywhere or do anything. I would lose my temper with the children and then cry because I knew they didn't deserve my impatience and irritability. My husband tried to be supportive and help but just couldn't understand what I was going through.

One day while cooking dinner and listening to the oprah show I heard Robin McGraw, Suzanne Summer and several doctors discussing the pros and cons of bioidentical hormones and for the first time felt like there might be some hope. I searched for a doctor in my area that could help me but I couldn't find one. I even e-mailed Oprah about my frustration. After several months went by I was just so desperate I decided to get a plane ticket and go to California to see the doctor from the Oprah show that had helped Robin McGraw. When I returned to Oprah's web-site to get the name of the doctor there was a link to body logic md and a participating doctor 2 hours away in Columbus, Ohio. I contacted them that day and started on the journey to get my life back. Once the necessary lab work was done to determine my hormone levels, I drove to Columbus and met with the doctor. I am now on bio identical hormones that address all of my symptoms as well as some nutritional supplements. I am now sleeping and the hot flashes and night sweats have disappeared. But most importantly, I am no longer so quick to anger and irritable. I have patience with my two girls and life is more harmonious. The joy has returned to my life. My libido is better, but not as good as my husband would like it to be. (They're never satisfied) the difference in my life has been dramatic.

-Roberta Flack

*A*t 53 years of age a chance visit to New York city to visit some dear friends in October 2006 would prove to be a defining moment in my life. As if the needs of those in my immediate care were not enough, I found myself serving as a director and volunteer in a relief organization that provided millions of dollars worth of relief and assistance to the devastated victims of 9-11 and hurricane katrina. Just a few shorts months prior to my visit I felt I was at the "top of my game." But stress, fatigue and over-commitment combined with age were taking a toll on my body and soul and mind, not to mention my wife and family. Chronic fatigue, depression, sleeplessness, and the inability to think clearly brought me to my necessary time away. My friends in nyc were alarmed at the radical changes in me. Their recommendation that I see Dr. Roger Garcia in columbus for an evaluation would become a major factor in my miraculous recovery to life. I had no idea that very high cortisol levels and extremely low* progesterone and testosterone were the primary culprits in my rapid regression from life. December 2006 was my turnaround month! After just one month of treatment under Dr. Garcia's care I began to come alive again. My mind began to clear, the depression lifted, chronic fatigue was replaced by energy and a renewed zest for life, and the sleeplessness was gone. My family and friends were amazed! Within two months I was ready to once again return to my life-calling and active lifestyle. Over the next year my weight would drop from 200 pounds to 170 as I once again had energy and drive to exercise and engage life head-on. Daily life and a busy, demanding schedule were no longer draining the life from me. I had received a new lease on life, thanks to the intervention of family and friends, and the introduction to my new life-long friends, Dr. Garcia and hormone replacement therapy. I now can look forward with joy to the future and my "aging to perfection."

-Jimmy Smith

I wanted to provide you with some feedack regarding my experience with Bodylogic md. I am a 42 year old African American male who has been involved in athletics most of my life. Over the past few years, I had noticed that my energy level was decreasing, I was more injury prone and just generally feeling lack luster. The most significant sign was that in the evening I would be so tired that I could not stay awake if I tried. There had been times when I would fall asleep midsentence. A friend actually had similar symptoms and as a favor I began researching options for him. My attention was brought to bodylogic md and I encouraged him to look into it. Another friend from the gym made the same recommendation. After, he informed me of his positive experience I decided to check it out for myself. I went to bodylogic soon after being advised by my primary physical that my cholesterol was at 250. Upon my first visit, I knew I was in the right place. Dr. Garcia spent more time with me and was more Informative about my health than my regular physician. I left the office with a new plan for eating, vitamin supplements, and testosterone replacement. After the first 3 months I have lost over 10 pounds, Maintained muscle, lowered my cholesterol to under 200 and can make It through an entire movie without falling asleep. I am glad I found Dr. Garcia

-John Jacobs

REFERENCES

Chapter 2 References

Connelly JE. The power of touch in clinical medicine. *Pharos Alpha Omega Alpha Honor Med Soc.* 2004 Spring;67(2):11-13.

Deutschman A. *Change or Die. Fast Company.* May 1, 2005. www.fastcompany.com/magazine/94/open_change-or-die.html?page=0%2C1. (Accessed November 10, 2009).

DiBiase R, and Gunnoe J. Gender and culture differences in touching behavior. *J Soc Psychol.* 2004 Feb;144(1):49-62.

Diego MA, Jones NA, and Field T. EEG in 1-week, 1-month and 3-month-old infants of depressed and non-depressed mothers. *Biol Psychol.* 2010 Jan;83(1):7-14.

Diggins K. The power of physical touch. *J Christ Nurs.* 2009 Apr-Jun;26(2):119.

Fascione J. Healing power of touch. *Elder Care.* 1995 Jan-Feb;7(1):19-21.

Felitti VJ. Adverse childhood experiences and adult health. *Acad Pediatr.* 2009 May-Jun;9(3):131-132.

Kemper KJ, Fletcher NB, Hamilton CA, and McLean TW. Impact of healing touch on pediatric oncology outpatients: pilot study. *J Soc Integr Oncol.* 2009 Winter;7(1):12-18.

Kuhn CM, and Schanberg SM. Responses to maternal separation: mechanisms and mediators. *Int J Dev Neurosci.* 1998 Jun-Jul;16(3-4):261-270.

Light KC, Grewen KM, and Amico JA. More frequent partner hugs and higher oxytocin levels are linked to lower blood pressure and heart rate in premenopausal women. *Biol Psychol.* 2005 Apr;69(1):5-21.

Mcgraw R. *What's Age Got To Do With It?* Nashville, Tennessee: Thomas Nelson, Inc., 2009.

Miles R, Cowan F, Glover V, Stevenson J, and Modi N. A controlled trial of skin-to-skin contact in extremely preterm infants. *Early Hum Dev.* 2006 Jul;82(7):447-455.

Perry B. The power of the simplest gesture. *Health Prog.* 2005 Sep-Oct;86(5):50-53.

Rosa L, Rosa E, Sarner L, and Barrett S. A close look at therapeutic touch. *JAMA.* 1998 Apr 1;279(13):1005-1110.

Snyder JR. Therapeutic touch and the terminally ill: healing power through the hands. *Am J Hosp Palliat Care.* 1997 Mar-Apr;14(2):83-87.

Ventegodt S, Morad M, and Merrick J. Clinical holistic medicine: classic art of healing or the therapeutic touch. *ScientificWorldJournal.* 2004 Mar 4;4:134-147.

Chapter 3 References

Abbott RD, Launer LJ, Rodriguez BL, Ross GW, Wilson PW, Masaki KH, Strozyk D, Curb JD, Yano K, Popper JS, and Petrovitch H. Serum estradiol and risk of stroke in elderly men. *Neurology.* 2007 Feb 20;68(8):563-568.

Andò S, De Amicis F, Rago V, Carpino A, Maggiolini M, Panno ML, and Lanzino M. Breast cancer: from estrogen to androgen receptor. *Mol Cell Endocrinol.* 2002 Jul 31;193(1-2):121-128.

Bansil S, Lee HJ, Jindal S, Holtz CR, and Cook SD. Correlation between sex hormones and magnetic resonance imaging lesions in multiple sclerosis. *Acta Neurol Scand.* 1999 Feb;99(2):91-94.

Bayliss RI, and Tunbridge WM. *Thyroid Disease: The Facts.* Third Edition. New York, NY: Oxford University Press, 1998.

Bergink EW, Kloosterboer HJ, vand an der Vies J. Oestrogen binding proteins in the female genital tract. *J Steroid Biochem.* 1984 Apr;20(4B):1057-1060.

Blanchard K, and Brill MB. *What Your Doctor May Not Tell You About Hypothyroidism; A Simple Plan for Extraordinary Results.* New York, NY: Wellness Central, 2004.

Blum M. Benefits of vaginal estriol cream combined with clonidine HCL for menopausal syndrome treatment. *Clin Exp Obstet Gynecol.* 1985;12(1-2):1-2.

Bradlow HL, Telang NT, Sepkovic DW, and Osborne MP. 2-hydroxyestrone: the 'good' estrogen. *J Endocrinol.* 1996 Sep;150 Suppl:S259-S265.

Brownstein D. *Iodine; Why You Need It, Why You Can't Live Without It.* West Bloomfield, Michigan: Medical Alternatives Press, 2008.

Brownstein D. *Overcoming Thyroid Disorders.* West Bloomfield, Michigan: Medical Alternatives Press, 2002.

Cedars MI, and Judd HL. Nonoral routes of estrogen administration. *Obstet Gynecol Clin North Am.* 1987 Mar;14(1):269-298.

Cutolo M, Seriolo B, Villaggio B, Pizzorni C, Craviotto C, and Sulli A. Androgens and estrogens modulate the immune and inflammatory responses in rheumatoid arthritis. *Ann N Y Acad Sci.* 2002 Jun;966:131-142.

de Lignieres B, Dennerstein L, and Backstrom T. Influence of route of administration on progesterone metabolism. *Maturitas.* 1995 Apr;21(3):251-257.

Debing E, Peeters E, Duquet W, Poppe K, Velkeniers B, and Van Den Brande P. Men with atherosclerotic stenosis of the carotid artery have lower testosterone levels compared with controls. *Int Angiol.* 2008 Apr;27(2):135-141.

Dew J, Eden J, Beller E, Magarey C, Schwartz P, Crea P, and Wren B. A cohort study of hormone replacement therapy given to women previously treated for breast cancer. *Climacteric.* 1998 Jun;1(2):137-142.

Dew JE, Wren BG, and Eden JA. A cohort study of topical vaginal estrogen therapy in women previously treated for breast cancer. *Climacteric.* 2003 Mar;6(1):45-52.

Dimitrakakis C, Zhou J, Wang J, Belanger A, LaBrie F, Cheng C, Powell D, and Bondy C. A physiologic role for testosterone in limiting estrogenic stimulation of the breast. *Menopause.* 2003 Jul-Aug;10(4):292-298.

Dong BJ, Hauck WW, Gambertoglio JG, et al. Bioequivalence of generic and brand-name levothyroxine products in the treatment of hypothyroidism. *JAMA.* 1997 Apr 16;277(15):1205-1213.

Dunajska K, Milewicz A, Szymczak J, Jȩdrzejuk D, Kuliczkowski W, Salomon P, and Nowicki P. Evaluation of sex hormone levels and some metabolic factors in men with coronary atherosclerosis. *Aging Male.* 2004 Sep;7(3):197-204.

Ficicioglu C, Gurbuz B, Tasdemir S, Yalti S, and Canova H. High local endometrial effect of vaginal progesterone gel. *Gynecol Endocrinol.* 2004 May;18(5):240-243.

Fishman J, and Martucci C. Biological properties of 16 alpha-hydroxyestrone: implications in estrogen physiology and pathophysiology. *J Clin Endocrinol* Metab. 1980 Sep;51(3):611-615.

Fitzpatrick LA, Pace C, and Wiita B. Comparison of regimens containing oral micronized progesterone or medroxyprogesterone acetate on quality of life in postmenopausal women: a cross-sectional survey. *J Womens Health Gend Based Med.* 2000 May;9(4):381-387.

Follingstad AH. Estriol, the forgotten estrogen? *JAMA.* 1978 Jan 2;239(1):29-30.

Fournier A, Berrino F, and Clavel-Chapelon F. Unequal risks for breast cancer associated with different hormone replacement therapies: results from the E3N cohort study. *Breast Cancer Res Treat.* 2008 Jan;107(1):103-111.

Fournier A, Berrino F, Riboli E, Avenel V, and Clavel-Chapelon F. Breast cancer risk in relation to different types of hormone replacement therapy in the E3N-EPIC cohort. *Int J Cancer.* 2005 Apr 10;114(3):448-454.

Friberg L, Drvota V, Bjelak AH, Eggertsen G, and Ahnve S. Association between increased levels of reverse triiodothyronine and mortality after acute myocardial infarction. *Am J Med.* 2001 Dec 15;111(9):699-703.

Gann PH, Hennekens CH, Longcope C, Verhoek-Oftedahl W, Grodstein F, and Stampfer MJ. A prospective study of plasma hormone levels, nonhormonal factors, and development of benign prostatic hyperplasia. *Prostate.* 1995 Jan;26(1):40-49.

Giton F, de la Taille A, Allory Y, Galons H, Vacherot F, Soyeux P, Abbou CC, Loric S, Cussenot O, Raynaud JP, and Fiet J. Estrone sulfate (E1S), a prognosis marker for tumor aggressiveness in prostate cancer (PCa). *J Steroid Biochem Mol Biol.* 2008 Mar;109(1-2):158-167.

Gordon ML. *The Clinical Application of Interventional Endocrinology.* Beverly Hills, CA: Phoenix Books, 2007.

Greenblatt RB, and Suran RR. Indications for hormonal pellets in the therapy of endocrine and gynecic disorders. *Am J Obstet Gynecol.* 1949 Feb;57(2):294-301.

Hak AE, Witteman JC, de Jong FH, Geerlings MI, Hofman A, and Pols HA. Low levels of endogenous androgens increase the risk of atherosclerosis in elderly men: the Rotterdam study. *J Clin Endocrinol Metab.* 2002 Aug;87(8):3632-3639.

Hamilton MA, and Stevenson LW. Thyroid hormone abnormalities in heart failure: possibilities for therapy. *Thyroid.* 1996 Oct;6(5):527-529.

Heimer G, and Englund D. Estriol: absorption after long-term vaginal treatment andgastrointestinal absorption as influenced by a meal. *Acta Obstet Gynecol Scand.* 1984;63(6):563-567.

Ho CK, Nanda J, Chapman KE, and Habib FK. Oestrogen and benign prostatic hyperplasia: effects on stromal cell proliferation and local formation from androgen. *J Endocrinol.* 2008 Jun;197(3):483-491.

Hofling M, Hirschberg AL, Skoog L, Tani E, Hägerström T, and von Schoultz B. Testosterone inhibits estrogen/progestogen-induced breast cell proliferation in postmenopausal women. *Menopause*. 2007 Mar-Apr;14(2):183-190.

Hogervorst E, Bandelow S, Combrinck M, and Smith AD. Low free testosterone is an independent risk factor for Alzheimer's disease. *Exp Gerontol*. 2004 Nov-Dec;39(11-12):1633-1639.

Hogervorst E, Combrinck M, and Smith AD. Testosterone and gonadotropin levels in men with dementia. *Neuro Endocrinol Lett*. 2003 Jun-Aug;24(3-4):203-208.

Jackson G. The importance of risk factor reduction in erectile dysfunction. *Curr Urol Rep*. 2007 Nov;8(6):463-466.

Janjua NR, Kongshoj B, Andersson AM, and Wulf HC. Sunscreens in human plasma and urine after repeated whole-body topical application. *J Eur Acad Dermatol Venereol*. 2008 Apr;22(4):456-461.

Jankowska EA, Rozentryt P, Ponikowska B, Hartmann O, Kustrzycka-Kratochwil D, Reczuch K, Nowak J, Borodulin-Nadzieja L, Polonski L, Banasiak W, Poole-Wilson PA, Anker SD, and Ponikowski P. Circulating estradiol and mortality in men with systolic chronic heart failure. *JAMA*. 2009 May 13;301(18):1892-1901.

Kabat GC, O'Leary ES, Gammon MD, Sepkovic DW, Teitelbaum SL, Britton JA, Terry MB, Neugut AI, and Bradlow HL. Estrogen metabolism and breast cancer. *Epidemiology*. 2006 Jan;17(1):80-88.

Keller PJ, Riedmann R, Fischer M, and Gerber C. Oestrogens, gonadotropins and prolactin after intra-vaginal administration of oestriol in post-menopausal women. *Maturitas*. 1981 Mar;3(1):47-53.

Khaw KT, Dowsett M, Folkerd E, Bingham S, Wareham N, Luben R, Welch A, and Day N. Endogenous testosterone and mortality due to all causes, cardiovascular disease, and cancer in men: European prospective investigation into cancer in Norfolk (EPIC-Norfolk) Prospective Population Study. *Circulation*. 2007 Dec 4;116(23):2694-2701.

Kim S, Liva SM, Dalal MA, Verity MA, and Voskuhl RR. Estriol ameliorates autoimmune demyelinating disease: implications for multiple sclerosis. *Neurology*. 1999 Apr 12;52(6):1230-1238.

Krieg M, Nass R, and Tunn S. Effect of aging on endogenous level of 5 alpha-dihydrotestosterone, testosterone, estradiol, and estrone in epithelium and stroma of normal and hyperplastic human prostate. *J Clin Endocrinol Metab*. 1993 Aug;77(2):375-381.

Krum H, and McMurray JJ. Statins and chronic heart failure: do we need a large-scale outcome trial? *J Am Coll Cardiol*. 2002 May 15;39(10):1567-1573.

Kuhl H. Pharmacology of estrogens and progestogens: influence of different routes of administration. *Climacteric*. 2005 Aug;8 Suppl 1:3-63.

Kuhn CM, and Schanberg SM. Responses to maternal separation: mechanisms and mediators. *Int J Dev Neurosci*. 1998 Jun-Jul;16(3-4):261-270.

Laaksonen DE, Niskanen L, Punnonen K, Nyyssönen K, Tuomainen TP, Salonen R, Rauramaa R, and Salonen JT. Sex hormones, inflammation and the metabolic syndrome: a population-based study. *Eur J Endocrinol*. 2003 Dec;149(6):601-608.

LeBlanc ES, Nielson CM, Marshall LM, Lapidus JA, Barrett-Connor E, Ensrud KE, Hoffman AR, Laughlin G, Ohlsson C, and Orwoll ES. Osteoporotic Fractures in Men Study Group. The effects of serum testosterone, estradiol, and sex hormone binding globulin levels on fracture risk in older men. *J Clin Endocrinol Metab*. 2009 Sep;94(9):3337-3346.

Lee J. *What Your Doctor May Not Tell You About Menopause*. New York, NY: Warner Books, 1996.

Levy T, Yairi Y, Bar-Hava I, Shalev J, Orvieto R, and Ben-Rafael Z. Pharmacokinetics of the progesterone-containing vaginal tablet and its use in assisted reproduction. *Steroids*. 2000 Oct-Nov;65(10-11):645-649.

Matsuda T, Abe H, and Suda K. Relation between benign prostatic hyperplasia and obesity and estrogen . *Rinsho Byori*. 2004 Apr;52(4):291-294.

Mattsson LA, and Cullberg G. Vaginal absorption of two estriol preparations. A comparative study in postmenopausal women. *Acta Obstet Gynecol Scand*. 1983;62(5):393-396.

McDougall IR. *Thyroid Disease in Clinical Practice*. New York, NY: Oxford University Press, 1992.

Mellström D, Vandenput L, Mallmin H, Holmberg AH, Lorentzon M, Odén A, Johansson H, Orwoll ES, Labrie F, Karlsson MK, Ljunggren O, and Ohlsson C. Older men with low serum estradiol and high serum SHBG have an increased risk of fractures. *J Bone Miner Res*. 2008 Oct;23(10):1552-1560.

Miller M. Hypothyroidism: Optimizing Medication with Slow-Release Compounded Thyroid Replacement. Int. *J. of Pharm. Compd*. 2005 July/August;9(4).

Milner M. Wilson's syndrome and T3 therapy: A clinical guide to safe and effective patient management. *Int. J. of Pharm Compd*. 1999;3(5):344-351.

Morgentaler A. *Testosterone for Life: Recharge Your Vitality, Sex Drive, Muscle Mass & Overall Health*. New York, NY: McGraw Hill, 2009.

Muller M, van den Beld AW, Bots ML, Grobbee DE, Lamberts SW, and van der Schouw YT. Endogenous sex hormones and progression of carotid atherosclerosis in elderly men. *Circulation*. 2004 May 4;109(17):2074-2079.

Natrajan PK, and Gambrell RD Jr. Estrogen replacement therapy in patients with early breast cancer. *Am J Obstet Gynecol*. 2002 Aug;187(2):289-294; discussion 294-295.

Newman TB, and Hulley SB. Carcinogenicity of lipid-lowering drugs. *JAMA*. 1996 Jan 3;275(1):55-60.

News conference at the American Heart Association Annual Meeting. November 17, 1994.

Osborne MP, Bradlow HL, Wong GY, and Telang NT. Upregulation of estradiol C16 alpha-hydroxylation in human breast tissue: a potential biomarker of breast cancer risk. *J Natl Cancer Inst*. 1993 Dec 1;85(23):1917-1920.

Prins GS, Huang L, Birch L, and Pu Y. The role of estrogens in normal and abnormal development of the prostate gland. *Ann N Y Acad Sci*. 2006 Nov;1089:1-13.

Prins GS, and Korach KS. The role of estrogens and estrogen receptors in normal prostate growth and disease. *Steroids*. 2008 Mar;73(3):233-244.

Punnonen R, Vilska S, Grönroos M, and Rauramo L. The vaginal absorption of oestrogens in post-menopausal women. *Maturitas*. 1980 Dec;2(4):321-326.

Refetoff S. Resistance to thyroid hormone. In Werner and Ingbar's *The Thyroid: A Fundamental and Clinical Text,* Seventh Edition, ed. Braverman LE and Utiger RE. Philadelphia, PA: Lippincott-Raven Publishers, 1996. 1032-1048.

Rennie, D. Thyroid Storm. *JAMA*. 1997 Apr 16;277(15):1238-1243.

Rich RL, Hoth LR, Geoghegan KF, Brown TA, LeMotte PK, Simons SP, Hensley P, and Myszka DG. Kinetic analysis of estrogen receptor/ligand interactions. *Proc Natl Acad Sci U S A*. 2002 Jun 25;99(13):8562-8567.

Rigg LA, Hermann H, and Yen SS. Absorption of estrogens from vaginal creams. *N Engl J Med*. 1978 Jan 26;298(4):195-197.

Rosenthal MS. *The Thyroid Sourcebook*. Fourth Edition. New York, NY: McGraw-Hill; 2000.

Ross R. Atherosclerosis--an inflammatory disease. *N Engl J Med*. 1999 Jan 14;340(2):115-126.

Schatz IJ, Masaki K, Yano K, Chen R, Rodriguez BL, and Curb JD. Cholesterol and all-cause mortality in elderly people from the Honolulu Heart Program: a cohort study. *Lancet*. 2001 Aug 4;358(9279):351-355.

Shibata Y, Ito K, Suzuki K, Nakano K, Fukabori Y, Suzuki R, Kawabe Y, Honma S, and Yamanaka H. Changes in the endocrine environment of the human prostate transition zone with aging: simultaneous quantitative analysis of prostatic sex steroids and comparison with human prostatic histological composition. *Prostate*. 2000 Jan;42(1):45-55.

Shippen E, and Fryer W. *Testostserone Syndrome; The Critical Factor for Energy, Health, & Sexuality- Reversing the Male Menopause*. New York, NY: M. Evans and Company, Inc., 1998.

Shomon MJ. *Mary Shomon's Thyroid Survey; A Comprehensive Patient-Oriented Quality of Life Survey.* www.thyroid.about.com/library/weekly/aa072101a.htm. (Accessed January 6, 2010).

Singh PB, Matanhelia SS, and Martin FL. A potential paradox in prostate adenocarcinoma progression: oestrogen as the initiating driver. *Eur J Cancer.* 2008 May;44(7):928-936.

Slagter MH, Gooren LJ, Scorilas A, Petraki CD, and Diamandis EP. Effects of long-term androgen administration on breast tissue of female-to-male transsexuals. *J Histochem Cytochem.* 2006 Aug;54(8):905-910.

Stanton A, and Tweed V. *Hormone Harmony; How to Balance Insulin, Cortisol, Thyroid, Estrogen, Progesterone, and Testosterone to Live Your Best Life.* Los Angeles, CA: Healthy Life Library, 2009.

Tang YJ, Lee WJ, Chen YT, Liu PH, Lee MC, and Sheu WH. Serum testosterone level and related metabolic factors in men over 70 years old. *J Endocrinol Invest.* 2007 Jun;30(6):451-458.

Temple T. *The Genius of China; 3,000 Years of Science, Discovery, and Invention.* New York, NY: Simon and Schuster, 1986.

Tivesten A, Vandenput L, Labrie F, Karlsson MK, Ljunggren O, Mellström D, and Ohlsson C. Low serum testosterone and estradiol predict mortality in elderly men. *J Clin Endocrinol Metab.* 2009 Jul;94(7):2482-2488.

Traish AM, Saad F, and Guay A. The dark side of testosterone deficiency: II. Type 2 diabetes and insulin resistance. *J Androl.* 2009 Jan-Feb;30(1):23-32.

Vooijs GP, and Geurts TB. Review of the endometrial safety during intravaginal treatment with estriol. *Eur J Obstet Gynecol Reprod Biol.* 1995 Sep;62(1):101-106.

Weiderpass E, Baron JA, Adami HO, Magnusson C, Lindgren A, Bergström R, Correia N, and Persson I. Low-potency oestrogen and risk of endometrial cancer: a case-control study. *Lancet.* 1999 May 29;353(9167):1824-1828.

Williams AB, and Williams RI. *Textbook of Endocrinology.* Philadelphia, PA: Saunders, 2003: 342.

Wilson ED. *Doctor's Manual for Wilson's Syndrome.* Third Edition. Lady Lake, FL: Muskeegee Medical Publishing Co.; 1997.

Wilson ED. *Wilson's Thyroid Syndrome: A Reversible Thyroid Problem.* Orlando, FL: Cornerstone Publishing Co; 1991.

Wranicz JK, Cygankiewicz I, Rosiak M, Kula P, Kula K, and Zareba W. The relationship between sex hormones and lipid profile in men with coronary artery disease. *Int J Cardiol.* 2005 May 11;101(1):105-110.

Wright JV, and Lenard L. *Stay Young and Sexy with Bio-Identical Hormone Replacement; The Science Explained.* Petaluma, CA: Smart Publications, 2010.

Zhou J, Ng S, Adesanya-Famuiya O, Anderson K, and Bondy CA. Testosterone inhibits estrogen-induced mammary epithelial proliferation and suppresses estrogen receptor expression. *FASEB J.* 2000 Sep;14(12):1725-1730.

Zhu BT, Han GZ, Shim JY, Wen Y, and Jiang XR. Quantitative structure-activity relationship of various endogenous estrogen metabolites for human estrogen receptor alpha and beta subtypes: Insights into the structural determinants favoring a differential subtype binding. *Endocrinology.* 2006 Sep;147(9):4132-4150.

Chapter 4 References

Ahmed A, and Tollefsbol T. Telomeres and telomerase: basic science implications for aging. *J Am Geriatr Soc.* 2001 Aug;49(8):1105-1109.

Ahmed N, and Thornalley PJ. Advanced glycation endproducts: what is the irrelevance to diabetic complications? *Diabetes Obes Metab.* 2007 May;9(3):233-245.

Amento EP. Vitamin D and the immune system. *Steroids.* 1987 Jan-Mar;49(1-3):55-72.

Appel LJ, Moore TJ, Obarzanek E, et al. A clinical trial of the effects of dietary patterns on blood pressure. DASH Collaborative Research Group. *N Engl J Med.* 1997;336:1117-1124.

Appleton N. *Suicide by Sugar; A Starling Look at Our #1 National Addiction.* Garden City Park, NY: Square One Publishers, 2009.

Auborn KJ, Fan S, Rosen EM, Goodwin L, Chandraskaren A, Williams DE, Chen D, and Carter TH. Indole-3-carbinol is a negative regulator of estrogen. *J Nutr.* 2003 Jul;133(7 Suppl):2470S-2475S.

Bell MC, Crowley-Nowick P, Bradlow HL, Sepkovic DW, Schmidt-Grimminger D, Howell P, Mayeaux EJ, Tucker A, Turbat-Herrera EA, and Mathis JM. Placebo-controlled trial of indole-3-carbinol in the treatment of CIN. *Gynecol Oncol.* 2000 Aug;78(2):123-129.

Bergman Jungeström M, Thompson LU, and Dabrosin C. Flaxseed and its lignans inhibit estradiol-induced growth, angiogenesis, and secretion of vascularendothelial growth factor in human breast cancer xenografts in vivo. *Clin Cancer Res.* 2007 Feb 1;13(3):1061-1067.

Bjelakovic G, Nikolova D, Gluud LL, Simonetti RG, and Gluud C. Mortality in randomized trials of antioxidant supplements for primary and secondary prevention: systematic review and meta-analysis. *JAMA.* 2007 Feb 28;297(8):842-857.

Bonkhoff H, and Fixemer T. [Implications of estrogens and their receptors for the development and progression of prostate cancer]. *Pathologe.* 2005 Nov;26(6):461-468.

Bradlow HL, Michnovicz JJ, Halper M, Miller DG, Wong GY, and Osborne MP. Long-term responses of women to indole-3-carbinol or a high fiber diet. *Cancer Epidemiol Biomarkers Prev.* 1994 Oct-Nov;3(7):591-595.

Bradlow HL, Sepkovic DW, Telang NT, and Osborne MP. Indole-3-carbinol. A novel approach to breast cancer prevention. *Ann N Y Acad Sci.* 1995 Sep 30;768:180-200.

Bradlow HL, Telang NT, Sepkovic DW, and Osborne MP. 2-hydroxyestrone: the 'good' estrogen. *J Endocrinol.* 1996 Sep;150 Suppl:S259-S265.

Brignall MS. Prevention and treatment of cancer with indole-3-carbinol. *Altern Med Rev.* 2001 Dec;6(6):580-589.

Brody JS, and Spira A. State of the art. Chronic obstructive pulmonary disease, inflammation, and lung cancer. *Proc Am Thorac Soc.* 2006 Aug;3(6):535-537.

Buettner D. *The Blue Zones; Lessons for Living Longer From the People Who've Lived the Longest.* Washington, DC: National Geographic, 2008.

Cameron NE, Gibson TM, Nangle MR, and Cotter MA. Inhibitors of advanced glycation end product formation and neurovascular dysfunction in experimental diabetes. *Ann N Y Acad Sci.* 2005 Jun;1043:784-792.

Campbell TC, and Campbell TM. *The China Study; Startling Implications for Diet, Weight Loss and Long Term Health.* Dallas, Texas: Benella Books, 2006.

Cannell J. *Vitamin D Newletter.* August 2006.

Cannell JJ, Vieth R, Umhau JC, Holick MF, Grant WB, Madronich S, Garland CF, and Giovannucci E. Epidemic influenza and vitamin D. *Epidemiol Infect.* 2006 Dec; 134(6):1129-1140.

Chel VG, Ooms ME, Popp-Snijders C, Pavel S, Schothorst AA, Meulemans CC, and Lips P. Ultraviolet irradiation corrects vitamin D deficiency and suppresses secondary hyperparathyroidism in the elderly. *J Bone Miner Res.* 1998 Aug;13(8):1238-1242.

Chen LH, Fang J, Li H, Demark-Wahnefried W, and Lin X. Enterolactone induces apoptosis in human prostate carcinoma LNCaP cells via a mitochondrial-mediated, caspase-dependent pathway. *Mol Cancer Ther.* 2007 Sep;6(9):2581-2890.

Cho E, Seddon JM, Rosner B, Willett WC, and Hankinson SE. Prospective study of intake of fruits, vegetables, vitamins, and carotenoids and risk of age-related maculopathy. *Arch Ophthalmol.* 2004;122:883–892.

Christen WG, Liu S, Glynn RJ, Gaziano JM, and Buring JE. Dietary carotenoids, vitamins C and E, and risk of cataract in women: A prospective study. *Arch Ophthalmol.* 2008;126:102–109.

Chrubasik JE, Roufogalis BD, Wagner H, and Chrubasik S. A comprehensive review on the stinging nettle effect and efficacy profiles. Part II: urticae radix. *Phytomedicine.* 2007 Aug;14(7-8):568-579.

Danaei G, Ding EL, Mozaffarian D, Taylor B, Rehm J, Murray CJ, and Ezzati M. The preventable causes of death in the United States: comparative risk assessment of dietary, lifestyle, and metabolic risk factors. *PLoS Med.* 2009 Apr 28;6(4):e1000058.

Després JP, and Lemieux I. Abdominal obesity and metabolic syndrome. *Nature.* 2006 Dec 14;444(7121):881-887.

Driscoll I, and Resnick SM. Testosterone and cognition in normal aging and Alzheimer's disease: an update. *Curr Alzheimer Res.* 2007 Feb;4(1):33-45.

Dukas L, Staehelin HB, Schacht E, and Bischoff HA. Better functional mobility in community-dwelling elderly is related to D-hormone serum levels and to daily calcium intake. *J Nutr Health Aging.* 2005 Sep-Oct;9(5):347-351.

Dusso AS, Brown AJ, and Slatopolsky E. Vitamin D. *Am J Physiol Renal Physiol.* 2005 Jul;289(1):F8-F28.

Esselstyn CB Jr, Ellis SG, Medendorp SV, and Crowe TD. A strategy to arrest and reverse coronary artery disease: a 5-year longitudinal study of a single physician's practice. *J Fam Pract.* 1995 Dec;41(6):560-568.

Evans BA, Griffiths K, and Morton MS. Inhibition of 5 alpha-reductase in genital skin fibroblasts and prostate tissue by dietary lignans and isoflavonoids. *J Endocrinol.* 1995 Nov;147(2):295-302.

Everitt AV, and Le Couteur DG. Life extension by calorie restriction in humans. *Ann N Y Acad Sci.* 2007 Oct;1114:428-433.

Fowke JH, Longcope C, and Hebert JR. Brassica vegetable consumption shifts estrogen metabolism in healthy postmenopausal women. *Cancer Epidemiol Biomarkers Prev.* 2000 Aug;9(8):773-779.

Franceschi C. Inflammaging as a major characteristic of old people: can it be prevented or cured? *Nutr Rev.* 2007 Dec;65(12 Pt 2):S173-S176.

Franceschi C, Capri M, Monti D, Giunta S, Olivieri F, Sevini F, Panourgia MP, Invidia L, Celani L, Scurti M, Cevenini E, Castellani GC, and Salvioli S. Inflammaging and anti-inflammaging: a systemic perspective on aging and longevity emerged from studies in humans. *Mech Ageing Dev.* 2007 Jan;128(1):92-105.

Fukino Y, Ikeda A, Maruyama K, Aoki N, Okubo T, and Iso H. Randomized controlled trial for an effect of green tea-extract powder supplementation on glucose abnormalities. *Eur J Clin Nutr.* 2008 Aug;62(8):953-960.

Giusti C, Gargiulo P. Advances in biochemical mechanisms of diabetic retinopathy. *Eur Rev Med Pharmacol Sci.* 2007 May-Jun;11(3):155-163.

Gonzales GF, Córdova A, Vega K, Chung A, Villena A, Góñez C, and Castillo S. Effect of Lepidium meyenii (MACA) on sexual desire and its absent relationship with serum testosterone levels in adult healthy men. *Andrologia.* 2002 Dec;34(6):367-372.

Guzik TJ, Mangalat D, and Korbut R. Adipocytokines - novel link between inflammation and vascular function? *J Physiol Pharmacol.* 2006 Dec;57(4):505-528.

He FJ, Nowson CA, and MacGregor GA. Fruit and vegetable consumption and stroke: meta-analysis of cohort studies. *Lancet.* 2006;367:320-326.

Head KA. Peripheral neuropathy: pathogenic mechanisms and alternative therapies. *Altern Med Rev.* 2006 Dec;11(4):294-329.

Hedelin M, Klint A, Chang ET, Bellocco R, Johansson JE, Andersson SO, Heinonen SM, Adlercreutz H, Adami HO, Grönberg H, and Bälter KA. Dietary phytoestrogen, serum enterolactone and risk of prostate cancer: the cancer prostate Sweden study (Sweden). *Cancer Causes Control.* 2006 Mar;17(2):169-180.

Heilbronn LK, de Jonge L, Frisard MI, DeLany JP, Larson-Meyer DE, Rood J, Nguyen T, Martin CK, Volaufova J, Most MM, Greenway FL, Smith SR, Deutsch WA, Williamson DA, Ravussin E, and Pennington CALERIE Team. Effect of 6-month calorie restriction on biomarkers of longevity, metabolic adaptation, and oxidative stress in overweight individuals: a randomized controlled trial. *JAMA.* 2006 Apr 5;295(13):1539-1548.

Hickie I, Naismith S, Ward PB, Turner K, Scott E, Mitchell P, Wilhelm K, and Parker G. Reduced hippocampal volumes and memory loss in patients with early- and late-onset depression. *Br J Psychiatry.* 2005 Mar;186:197-202.

Ho GH, Luo XW, Ji CY, Foo SC, and Ng EH. Urinary 2/16 alpha-hydroxyestrone ratio: correlation with serum insulin-like growth factor binding protein-3 and apotential biomarker of breast cancer risk. *Ann Acad Med Singapore.* 1998 Mar;27(2):294-299.

Holick MF. The vitamin D epidemic and its health consequences. *J Nutr.* 2005 Nov;135(11):2739S-2748S.

Hung HC, Joshipura KJ, Jiang R, et al. Fruit and vegetable intake and risk of major chronic disease. *J Natl Cancer Inst.* 2004;96:1577–1584

Hutchins AM, Martini MC, Olson BA, Thomas W, and Slavin JL. Flaxseed consumption influences endogenous hormone concentrations in postmenopausal women. *Nutr Cancer.* 2001;39(1):58-65.

Itomura M, Hamazaki K, Sawazaki S, Kobayashi M, Terasawa K, Watanabe S, and Hamazaki T. The effect of fish oil on physical aggression in schoolchildren—a randomized, double-blind, placebo-controlled trial. *J Nutr Biochem.* 2005 Mar;16(3):163-171.

Jellinck PH, Forkert PG, Riddick DS, Okey AB, Michnovicz JJ, and Bradlow HL. Ah receptor binding properties of indole carbinols and induction of hepatic estradiol hydroxylation. *Biochem Pharmacol.* 1993 Mar 9;45(5):1129-1136.

Johansson S, and Melhus H. Vitamin A antagonizes calcium response to vitamin D in man. *J Bone Miner Res.* 2001 Oct;16(10):1899-1905.

Kabat GC, Chang CJ, Sparano JA, Sepkovie DW, Hu XP, Khalil A, Rosenblatt R, and Bradlow HL. Urinary estrogen metabolites and breast cancer: a case-control study. *Cancer Epidemiol Biomarkers Prev.* 1997 Jul;6(7):505-509.

Kabat GC, O'Leary ES, Gammon MD, Sepkovic DW, Teitelbaum SL, Britton JA, Terry MB, Neugut AI, and Bradlow HL. Estrogen metabolism and breast cancer. *Epidemiology.* 2006 Jan;17(1):80-88.

Kall MA, Vang O, and Clausen J. Effects of dietary broccoli on human drug metabolising activity. *Cancer Lett.* 1997 Mar 19;114(1-2):169-170.

Karachalias N, Babaei-Jadidi R, Ahmed N, and Thornalley PJ. Accumulation of fructosyl-lysine and advanced glycation end products in the kidney, retina and peripheral nerve of streptozotocin-induced diabetic rats. *Biochem Soc Trans.* 2003 Dec;31(Pt 6):1423-1425.

Kavanaugh CJ, Trumbo PR, and Ellwood KC. The U.S. Food and Drug Administration's evidence-based review for qualified health claims: tomatoes, lycopene, and cancer. *J Natl Cancer Inst.* 2007;99:1074–1085.

Koyama H, Yamamoto H, and Nishizawa Y. RAGE and soluble RAGE: potential therapeutic targets for cardiovascular diseases. *Mol Med.* 2007 Nov-Dec;13(11-12):625-635.

Krazeisen A, Breitling R, Möller G, and Adamski J. Phytoestrogens inhibit human 17beta-hydroxysteroid dehydrogenase type 5. *Mol Cell Endocrinol.* 2001 Jan 22;171(1-2):151-162.

Krinsky NI, Landrum JT, and Bone RA. Biologic mechanisms of the protective role of lutein and zeaxanthin in the eye. *Annu Rev Nutr.* 2003;23:171–201.

Lehman TD, and Ortwerth BJ. Inhibitors of advanced glycation end product-associated protein cross-linking. *Biochim Biophys Acta.* 2001 Feb 14;1535(2):110-119.

Lembo A, and Camilleri M. Chronic constipation. *N Engl J Med.* 2003;349:1360–1368.

Linus Pauling Institute. Indole-3-Carbinol. *http://lpi.oregonstate.edu/infocenter/* phytochemicals/i3c/. Oregon State University. (Accessed March 4, 2010).

Lord RS, Bongiovanni B, and Bralley JA. Estrogen metabolism and the diet-cancer connection: rationale for assessing the ratio of urinary hydroxylated estrogen metabolites. *Altern Med Rev.* 2002 Apr;7(2):112-129.

MacLaughlin J, and Holick MF. Aging decreases the capacity of human skin to produce vitamin D3. *J Clin Invest.* 1985 Oct;76(4):1536-1538.

Maroon J, and Bost J. *Fish Oil: The Natural Anti-Inflammatory.* Laguna Beach, CA: Basic Health Publications, 2006.

May E, Asadullah K, and Zügel U. Immunoregulation through 1,25-dihydroxyvitamin D3 and its analogs. *Curr Drug Targets Inflamm Allergy.* 2004 Dec;3(4):377-393.

McCann JC, and Ames BN. Is docosahexaenoic acid, an n-3 long-chain polyunsaturated fatty acid, required for development of normal brain function? An overview of evidence from cognitive and behavioral tests in humans and animals. *Am J Clin Nutr.* 2005 Aug;82(2):281-295.

McCann SE, Muti P, Vito D, Edge SB, Trevisan M, Freudenheim JL. Dietary lignan intakes and risk of pre- and postmenopausal breast cancer. *Int J Cancer.* 2004 Sep 1;111(3):440-443.

Menshikova EV, Ritov VB, Toledo FG, Ferrell RE, Goodpaster BH, and Kelley DE. Effects of weight loss and physical activity on skeletal muscle mitochondrial function in obesity. *Am J Physiol Endocrinol Metab.* 2005 Apr;288(4):E818-E825.

Michnoviez JJ, and Bradlow HL. Altered estrogen metabolism and excretion in humans following consumption of indole-3-carbinol. *Nutr Cancer.* 1991;16 (1):59-66.

Michnoviez JJ, and Bradlow HL. Induction of estradiol metabolism by dietary indole-3-carbinol in humans. *J Natl Cancer Inst.* 1990;82(11):947-949.

Moon YJ, Wang X, and Morris ME. Dietary flavonoids: effects on xenobiotic and carcinogen metabolism. *Toxicol In Vitro.* 2006 Mar;20(2):187-210.

Nagpal S, Na S, and Rathnachalam R. Noncalcemic actions of vitamin D receptor ligands. *Endocr Rev.* 2005 Aug;26(5):662-687.

Need AG, Morris HA, Horowitz M, and Nordin C. Effects of skin thickness, age, body fat, and sunlight on serum 25-hydroxyvitamin D. *Am J Clin Nutr.* 1993 Dec;58(6):882-885.

Norris JM, Yin X, Lamb MM, Barriga K, Seifert J, Hoffman M, Orton HD, Barón AE, Clare-Salzler M, Chase HP, Szabo NJ, Erlich H, Eisenbarth GS, and Rewers M. Omega-3 polyunsaturated fatty acid intake and islet autoimmunity in children at increased risk for type 1 diabetes. *JAMA.* 2007 Sep 26;298(12):1420-1428.

Ordovas J. Diet/genetic interactions and their effects on inflammatory markers. *Nutr Rev.* 2007 Dec;65(12 Pt 2):S203-S207.

Ornish D, Brown SE, Scherwitz LW, Billings JH, Armstrong WT, Ports TA, McLanahan SM, Kirkeeide RL, Brand RJ, and Gould KL. Can lifestyle changes reverse coronary heart disease? The Lifestyle Heart Trial. *Lancet.* 1990 Jul21;336(8708):129-133.

Ornish D, Lin J, Daubenmier J, Weidner G, Epel E, Kemp C, Magbanua MJ, Marlin R, Yglecias L, Carroll PR, and Blackburn EH. Increased telomerase activity and comprehensive lifestyle changes: a pilot study. *Lancet Oncol.* 2008 Nov;9(11):1048-1057.

Perlmutter D, and Coleman C. *Raise a Smarter Child by Kindergarten; Raise IQ by Up to Thirty Points and Turn On Your Childs Smart Genes.* New York, NY: Broadway Books, 2006.

Persson I. The risk of endometrial and breast cancer after estrogen treatment. A review of epidemiological studies. *Acta Obstet Gynecol Scand* Suppl. 1985;130:59-66.

Raffoul JJ, Guo Z, Soofi A, and Heydari AR. Caloric restriction and genomic stability. *J Nutr Health Aging.* 1999;3(2):102-110.

Regan E, Flannelly J, Bowler R, Tran K, Nicks M, Carbone BD, Glueck D, Heijnen H, Mason R, and Crapo J. Extracellular superoxide dismutase and oxidant damage in osteoarthritis. *Arthritis Rheum.* 2005 Nov;52(11):3479-3491.

Saarinen NM, Wärri A, Mäkelä SI, Eckerman C, Reunanen M, Ahotupa M, Salmi SM, Franke AA, Kangas L, and Santti R. Hydroxymatairesinol, a novel enterolactone precursor with antitumor properties from coniferous tree (Picea abies). *Nutr Cancer.* 2000;36(2):207-216.

Sanz J, Moreno PR, and Fuster V. Update on advances in atherothrombosis. *Nat Clin Pract Cardiovasc Med.* 2007 Feb;4(2):78-89.

Schneider J, Kinne D, Fracchia A, Pierce V, Anderson KE, Bradlow HL, and Fishman J. Abnormal oxidative metabolism of estradiol in women with breast cancer. *Proc Natl Acad Sci U S A.* 1982 May;79(9):3047-3051.

Schupp N, Schmid U, Heidland A, and Stopper H. New approaches for the treatment of genomic damage in end-stage renal disease. *J Ren Nutr.* 2008 Jan;18(1):127-133.

Steiner MS, Raghow S. Antiestrogens and selective estrogen receptor modulators reduce prostate cancer risk. *World J Urol.* 2003 May;21(1):31-36.

Suji G, and Sivakami S. DNA damage during glycation of lysine by methylglyoxal: assessment of vitamins in preventing damage. *Amino Acids.* 2007 Nov;33(4):615-621.

Telang NT, Suto A, Wong GY, Osborne MP, and Bradlow HL. Induction by estrogen metabolite 16 alpha-hydroxyestrone of genotoxic damage and aberrant proliferation in mouse mammary epithelial cells. *J Natl Cancer Inst.* 1992 Apr 15;84(8):634-638.

Terry P, Wolk A, Persson I, and Magnusson C. Brassica vegetables and breast cancer risk. *JAMA.* 2001 Jun 20;285(23):2975-2977.

Thornalley PJ. Glycation in diabetic neuropathy: characteristics, consequences, causes, and therapeutic options. *Int Rev Neurobiol.* 2002;50:37-57.

Trump DL, Deeb KK, and Johnson CS. Vitamin D: considerations in the continued development as an agent for cancer prevention and therapy. *Cancer J.* 2010 Jan-Feb;16(1):1-9.

2005 Dietary Guidelines for Americans. Center for Nutrition Policy and Promotion, U.S. Department of Agriculture.

Ursin G, London S, Stanczyk FZ, Gentzschein E, Paganini-Hill A, Ross RK, and Pike MC. Urinary 2-hydroxyestrone/16alpha-hydroxyestrone ratio and risk of breast cancer in postmenopausal women. *J Natl Cancer Inst.* 1999 Jun 16;91(12):1067-1072.

Vasdev S, Gill V, and Singal P. Role of advanced glycation end products in hypertension and atherosclerosis: therapeutic implications. *Cell Biochem Biophys.* 2007;49(1):48-63.

Wang C, Mäkelä T, Hase T, Adlercreutz H, and Kurzer MS. Lignans and flavonoids inhibit aromatase enzyme in human preadipocytes. *J Steroid Biochem Mol Biol.* 1994 Aug;50(3-4):205-212.

Wong GY, Bradlow L, Sepkovic D, Mehl S, Mailman J, and Osborne MP. Dose-ranging study of indole-3-carbinol for breast cancer prevention. *J Cell Biochem Suppl.*1997;28-29:111-116.

Wright JV, and Lenard L. *Stay Young and Sexy with Bio-Identical Hormone Replacement; The Science Explained.* Petaluma, CA: Smart Publications, 2010.

Wright RJ. Make no bones about it: increasing epidemiologic evidence links vitamin D to pulmonary function and COPD. *Chest.* 2005 Dec;128(6):3781-3783.

Yeap BB, Almeida OP, Hyde Z, Norman PE, Chubb SA, Jamrozik K, and Flicker L. In men older than 70 years, total testosterone remains stable while free testosterone declines with age. The Health in Men Study. *Eur J Endocrinol.* 2007 May;156(5):585-594.

Yee YK, Chintalacharuvu SR, Lu J, and Nagpal S. Vitamin D receptor modulators for inflammation and cancer. *Mini Rev Med Chem.* 2005 Aug;5(8):761-778.

Yehuda S, Rabinovitz S, and Mostofsky DI. Essential fatty acids and the brain: from infancy to aging. *Neurobiol Aging.* 2005 Dec;26 Suppl 1:98-102.

Yehuda S, Rabinovitz S, and Mostofsky DI. Nutritional deficiencies in learning and cognition. *J Pediatr Gastroenterol Nutr.* 2006 Dec;43 Suppl 3:S22-S25.

Zumoff B. Hormonal profiles in women with breast cancer. *Obstet Gynecol Clin North Am.* 1994 Dec;21(4):751-772.

Chapter 5 References

Benor DJ, Ledger K, Toussaint L, Hett G, and Zaccaro D. Pilot study of emotional freedom techniques, wholistic hybrid derived from eye movement desensitization and reprocessing and emotional freedom technique, and cognitive behavioral therapy for treatment of test anxiety in university students. Explore (NY). 2009.

Brown DP. The Energy Body and Its Functions: Immunosurveillance, Longevity, and Regeneration. *Ann N Y Acad Sci.* 2007 Sep 28.

Brown RP, and Gerbarg PL. Yoga breathing, meditation, and longevity. *Ann N Y Acad Sci.* 2009 Aug;1172:54-62.

Buettner D. *The Blue Zones; Lessons for Living Longer From the People Who've Lived the Longest.* Washington, DC: National Geographic, 2008.

Bushell WC, and Theise ND. Toward a unified field of study: longevity, regeneration, and protection of health through meditation and related practices. *Ann N Y Acad Sci.* 2009 Aug;1172:5-19.

Drapeau J, Gosselin N, Gagnon L, Peretz I, and Lorrain D. Emotional recognition from face, voice, and music in dementia of the Alzheimer type. *Ann N Y Acad Sci.* 2009 Jul;1169:342-345.

Hyman M. *The UltraMind Solution; Fix Your Broken Brain by Healing Your Body First.* New York, NY: Scribner, 2009.

Lupien SJ, Maheu F, Tu M, Fiocco A, and Schramek TE. The effects of stress and stress hormones on human cognition: Implications for the field of brain and cognition. *Brain Congn.* 2007 Dec; 65 (3): 209-37.

Martarelli D, Cocchioni M, Scuri S, and Pompei P. Diaphragmatic Breathing Reduces Exercise-induced Oxidative Stress. *Evid Based Complement Alternat Med.* 2009 Oct 29.

Pruessner JC, Baldwin MW, Dedovic K, Renwick R, Mahani NK, Lord C, Meaney M, and Lupien S. Self-esteem, locus of control, hippocampal volume, and cortisol regulation in young and old adulthood. *Neuroimage.* 2005 Dec;28(4):815-826.

Sapolsky RM. *Why Zebras Don't Get Ulcers.* New York, NY: Henry Holt and Company, 2004.

Schultz PW. *The Moral Call of the Wild. Scientific American.* December 1, 2009. http://www.scientificamerica.com/article.cfm?is=moral-call-of-the-wild. (Accessed January 28, 2010).

Shealy N, and Church D. Soul Medicine; *Awakening Your Inner Blueprint for Abundant Health and Energy.* Santa Rosa, CA; Energy Psychology Press, 2008.

Sloan RP, McCreath H, Tracey KJ, Sidney S, Liu K, and Seeman T. RR intervalvariability is inversely related to inflammatory markers: the CARDIA study. *Mol Med.* 2007 Mar-Apr;13(3-4):178-184.

Starkman MN, Gebarski SS, Berent S, and Schteingart DE. Hippocampal formation volume, memory dysfunction, and cortisol levels in patients with Cushing's syndrome. *Biol Psychiatry.* 1992 Nov 1;32(9):756-765.

Starkman MN, Giordani B, Gebarski SS, Berent S, Schork MA, Schteingart DE. Decrease in cortisol reverses human hippocampal atrophy following treatment of Cushing's disease. *Biol Psychiatry.* 1999 Dec 15;46(12):1595-1602.

Uno H, Eisele S, Sakai A, Shelton S, Baker E, DeJesus O, and Holden J. Neurotoxicity of glucocorticoids in the primate brain. *Horm Behav.* 1994 Dec;28(4):336-348.

Vanstone AD, and Cuddy LL. Musical memory in Alzheimer disease. *Neuropsychol Dev Cogn B Aging Neuropsychol Cogn.* 2010 Jan;17(1):108-128.

Vanstone AD, Cuddy LL, Duffin JM, and Alexander E. Exceptional preservation of memory for tunes and lyrics: case studies of amusia, profound deafness, and Alzheimer's disease. *Ann N Y Acad Sci.* 2009 Jul;1169:291-294.

Viktor Frankl - Holocaust Survivor and Famous Author/Psychoanalyst. www.rjgeib.com/thoughts/frankl/frankl.html. (Accessed February 27, 2010).

Weinstein N, Przybylski AK, and Ryan RM. Can nature make us more caring? Effects of immersion in nature on intrinsic aspirations and generosity. *Pers Soc Psychol Bull*. 2009 Oct;35(10):1315-1329.

Chapter 6 References

Bacon CG, Mittleman MA, Kawachi I, Giovannucci E, Glasser DB, and Rimm EB. Sexual function in men older than 50 years of age: results from the health professionals follow-up study. *Ann Intern Med*. 2003 Aug 5;139(3):161-168.

Berchtold NC, Castello N, and Cotman CW. Exercise and time-dependent benefits to learning and memory. *Neuroscience*. 2010 May 19;167(3):588-597.

Bravata DM, Smith-Spangler C, Sundaram V, Gienger AL, Lin N, Lewis R, Stave CD, Olkin I, and Sirard JR. Using pedometers to increase physical activity and improve health: a systematic review. *JAMA*. 2007 Nov 21;298(19):2296-2304.

Buettner D. *The Blue Zones; Lessons for Living Longer From the People Who've Lived the Longest*. Washington, DC: National Geographic, 2008.

Bushell WC, and Theise ND. Toward a unified field of study: longevity, regeneration, and protection of health through meditation and related practices. *Ann N Y Acad Sci*. 2009 Aug;1172:5-19.

Flint-Wagner HG, Lisse J, Lohman TG, Going SB, Guido T, Cussler E, Gates D, and Yocum DE. Assessment of a sixteen-week training program on strength, pain, and function in rheumatoid arthritis patients. *J Clin Rheumatol*. 2009 Jun;15(4):165-171.

Griesbach GS, Hovda DA, Molteni R, Wu A, Gomez-Pinilla F. Voluntary exercise following traumatic brain injury: brain-derived neurotrophic factor upregulation and recovery of function. *Neuroscience*. 2004;125(1):129-139.

Jackson G. The importance of risk factor reduction in erectile dysfunction. *Curr Urol Rep*. 2007 Nov;8(6):463-466.

Klepper SE. Effects of an eight-week physical conditioning program on disease signs and symptoms in children with chronic arthritis. *Arthritis Care Res*. 1999 Feb;12(1):52-60.

Landi F, Russo A, Cesari M, Pahor M, Liperoti R, Danese P, Bernabei R, and Onder G. Walking one hour or more per day prevented mortality among older persons: results from ilSIRENTE study. *Prev Med*. 2008 Oct;47(4):422-426.

Lee IM, and Paffenbarger RS Jr. Physical activity and stroke incidence: the Harvard Alumni Health Study. *Stroke*. 1998 Oct;29(10):2049-2054.

Manini TM, Everhart JE, Patel KV, Schoeller DA, Colbert LH, Visser M, Tylavsky F, Bauer DC, Goodpaster BH, and Harris TB. Daily activity energy expenditure and mortality among older adults. *JAMA*. 2006 Jul 12;296(2):171-179.

Mayo Clinic Staff. Depression and Anxiety: Exercise Eases Symptoms. *http://www.mayclinic.com/health/depression/depression-and-exercise/MH00043*. (Accessed February 24, 2010).

McGavock JM, Hastings JL, Snell PG, McGuire DK, Pacini EL, Levine BD, and Mitchell JH. A forty-year follow-up of the Dallas Bed Rest and Training study: the effect of age on the cardiovascular response to exercise in men. *J Gerontol A Biol Sci Med Sci*. 2009 Feb;64(2):293-299.

McGuire DK, Levine BD, Williamson JW, Snell PG, Blomqvist CG, Saltin B, and Mitchell JH. A 30-year follow-up of the Dallas Bedrest and Training Study: II. Effect of age on cardiovascular adaptation to exercise training. *Circulation*. 2001 Sep 18;104(12):1358-1366.

Meyerhardt JA, Giovannucci EL, Ogino S, Kirkner GJ, Chan AT, Willett W, and Fuchs CS. Physical activity and male colorectal cancer survival. *Arch Intern Med*. 2009 Dec 14;169(22):2102-2108.

Paffenbarger RS Jr, Hyde RT, Hsieh CC, and Wing AL. Physical activity, other life-style patterns, cardiovascular disease and longevity. *Acta Med Scand Suppl*. 1986;711:85-91.

Rolland Y, Abellan van Kan G, and Vellas B. Physical activity and Alzheimer's disease: from prevention to therapeutic perspectives. *J Am Med Dir Assoc*. 2008 Jul;9(6):390-405.

Rolland Y, van Kan GA, and Vellas B. Healthy brain aging: role of exercise and physical activity. *Clin Geriatr Med*. 2010 Feb;26(1):75-87.

Stessman J, Hammerman-Rozenberg R, Cohen A, Ein-Mor E, and Jacobs JM. Physical activity, function, and longevity among the very old. *Arch Intern Med*. 2009 Sep 14;169(16):1476-1483.

Tudor-Locke C, and Lutes L. Why do pedometers work?: a reflection upon the factors related to successfully increasing physical activity. *Sports Med*. 2009;39(12):981-993.

Chapter 7 References

Amen DG. *Magnificent Mind at Any Age; Natural Ways to Unleash Your Brain's Maximum Potential*. New York, NY: Three Rivers Press, 2008.

Anda RF, Dong M, Brown DW, Felitti VJ, Giles WH, Perry GS, Valerie EJ, and Dube SR. The relationship of adverse childhood experiences to a history of premature death of family members. *BMC Public Health*. 2009 Apr 16;9:106.

Boekhoorn SS, Vingerling JR, Uitterlinden AG, Van Meurs JB, van Duijn CM, Pols HA, Hofman A, and de Jong PT. Estrogen receptor alpha gene polymorphisms associated with incident aging macula disorder. *Invest Ophthalmol Vis Sci*. 2007 Mar;48(3):1012-1017.

Buettner D. *The Blue Zones;* Lessons for Living Longer From the People Who've Lived the Longest. Washington, DC: National Geographic, 2008.

Church D. *The Genie in Your Genes.* Santa Rosa, CA: Elite Books, 2007.

Clement, BR. *Supplements Exposed; The Truth They Don't Want You to Know About Vitamins, Minerals, and Their Effects on Your Health.* Franklin Lakes, NJ: Career Press, 2010.

Colbert D. *Toxic Relief.* Lake Mary, FL: Siloam, 2001.

Driscoll I, and Resnick SM. Testosterone and cognition in normal aging and Alzheimer's disease: an update. *Curr Alzheimer Res.* 2007 Feb;4(1):33-45.

Felitti VJ. Adverse childhood experiences and adult health. *Acad Pediatr.* 2009 May-Jun;9(3):131-132.

Futterman AD, Kemeny ME, Shapiro D, and Fahey JL. Immunological and physiological changes associated with induced positive and negative mood. *Psychosomatic Medicine.* Vol 56, Issue 6:499-511.

Hahn RA. The nocebo phenomenon: concept, evidence, and implications for public health. *Prev Med.* 1997 Sep-Oct;26(5 Pt 1):607-611.

Hickie I, Naismith S, Ward PB, Turner K, Scott E, Mitchell P, Wilhelm K, and Parker G. Reduced hippocampal volumes and memory loss in patients with early- and late-onset depression. *Br J Psychiatry.* 2005 Mar;186:197-202.

Hirst M, and Marra MA. Epigenetics and human disease. *Int J Biochem Cell Biol.* 2009 Jan;41(1):136-146.

Holder D. *"Does the Fear of Dying Become a Self-fulfilling Prophecy for People?" Oakland Tribune.* Nov 12, 2007.

Jere D. "Learning to Love Growing Old - Fear of aging speeds the very decline we dread most." *Psychology Today.* Sep/Oct 94.

Labott SM, Ahleman S, Wolever ME, and Martin RB. The physiological and psychological effects of the expression and inhibition of emotion. University of Toledo, Ohio. *Psychosomatic Medicine.* Vol 56, Issue 6:499-511.

Lipton B. http://www.brucelipton.com

Lipton B. *The Biology of Belief.* New York City, NY: Hay House, Inc., 2008.

Loop MJ. *"The Secret Law of Attraction Makes you Healthy and Rich."* March 7, 2008. http://healthandfitnessworld.wordpress.com/2008/03/07/the-secret-law-of-attraction-makes-you-healthy-and-rich/

MacMaster FP, and Kusumakar V. Hippocampal volume in early onset depression. *BMC Med.* 2004 Jan 29;2:2.

Ornish D, Lin J, Daubenmier J, Weidner G, Epel E, Kemp C, Magbanua MJ, Marlin R, Yglecias L, Carroll PR, and Blackburn EH. Increased telomerase activity and comprehensive lifestyle changes: a pilot study. *Lancet Oncol.* 2008 Nov;9(11):1048-1057.

Pert C. Molecules of Emotion. http://candacepert.com

Pert CB, Ruff MR, Weber RJ, and Herkenham M. Neuropeptides and their receptors: a psychosomatic network. *Journal of Immunol.* 1985 Aug;135(2 Suppl):820-826.

Quinlan J. *"Cell Consciousness – Proves Mind Over Matter."* http://www.infinityinst.com/article...

Rossi EL. *The Psychobiology of Gene Expression.* New York, NY: W.W. Norton & Company, 2002.

Rubin J. *The Great Physician Rx for Health and Wellness; Seven Keys to Unlock Yours* Scheinman PL. Prevalence of fragrance allergy. *Dermatology.* 2002;205(1):98-102.

Shealy N, and Church D. Soul Medicine; *Awakening Your Inner Blueprint for Abundant Health and Energy.* Santa Rosa, CA; Energy Psychology Press, 2008.

Sloan RP, Shapiro PA, Bagiella E, Boni SM, Paik M, Bigger JT Jr, Steinman RC, and Gorman JM. *Effect of mental stress throughout the day on cardiac autonomic control.* Behavioral Medicine Program, Columbia-Presbyterian Medical Center, New York, NY.

University of Rochester Medical Center (2005, October 10). *"I Think, Therefore I Fall." Science Daily.* http://www.sciencedaily.com/release...

Vinding T, and Nielsen NV. Retinopathy caused by treatment with tamoxifen in low dosage. *Acta Ophthalmol (Copenh).* 1983 Feb;61(1):45-50.

Weil A. Attitude is everything in aging. *Andrew Weil's Self Healing Newsletter.* September 2006, p.1.

Weinhold B. Epigenetics: the science of change. *Environ Health Perspect.* 2006 Mar;114(3):A160-A167.

Chapter 8 References

The American Academy of Environment Medicine. Genetically Modified Foods Position Paper. May 8, 2009. Genetically Modified Foods Position Paper: The American Academy. *www.aaemonline.org/gmopost.html.* (Accessed March 28, 2010).

The American Academy of Environmental Medicine Calls for Immediate Moratorium on Genetically Modified Foods. *www.aaemonline.org/gmopressrelease.html.* (Accessed March 29, 2010).

American Industrial Hygiene Association 2004. *Biological Monitoring: A Practical Field Manual.* Fairfax, VA: AIHA Press.

Baker N. *The Body Toxic, How the Hazardous Chemistry of Everyday Things Threatens Our Health and Well-being.* New York, NY: North Point Press, 2008.

Bisphenol-A website. www.ewg.org/tap-water/home. (Accessed April 6, 2010).

Blanc PD. *How Everyday Products Make People Sick; Toxins at Home and in the Workplace.* Berkeley and Los Angeles, California: University of California Press, 2009.

Blanchard K, and Brill MB. *What Your Doctor May Not Tell You About Hypothyroidism; A Simple Plan for Extraordinary Results.* New York, NY: Wellness Central, 2004.

Boas M, Feldt-Rasmussen U, Skakkebaek N, and Main K. Environmental chemicals and thyroid function *Eur J Endocrinol.* 2006 154:599–611.

Bryson C. *The Fluoride Deception.* New York: Seven Stories Press, 2004.

Carlson R. *Silent Spring.* Houghton Mifflin, 1962.

Casals M. Holistic Wellness. *Trihalomethanes Contaminants in Drinking Water. March 3, 2010. holisticwellnessshow.com/trihalomethanes-contaminants-in-drinking-water.* (Accessed April 5, 2010).

Centers for Disease Control. 2008. Fourth National Report on Human Exposure to Environmental Chemicals. Atlanta, GA: National Center for Environmental Health, Centers for Disease Control and Prevention. http://www.cdc.gov/exposurereport/. (Accessed March 16, 2010).

Centers for Disease Control and Prevention. National Biomonitoring Program. www.cdc.gov/biomonitoring (Accessed March 15, 2010).

Clean Air Act of 1990. Public Law 101–549.

Cone M. *Silent Snow: The Slow Poisoning of the Arctic.* New York, NY: Grove Press, 2005.

de Groot AC, and Frosch PJ. Adverse reactions to fragrances: A clinical review. *Contact Dermatitis.* 1997;36(2):57-86.

DeCaprio AP. Biomarkers: coming of age for environmental health and risk assessment. *Environ Sci Tech.* 1997;31:1837-1848.

Duncan DE. The pollution within. *Nat Geog* 2006 Oct;122.

Duty SM, Calafat AM, Silva MJ, Brock JW, Ryan L, Chen Z, et al. The relationship between environmental exposure to phthalates and computer-aided sperm analysis motion parameters. *Journal of andrology* 2004;25(2):293-302.

Duty SM, Silva MJ, Barr DB, Brock JW, Ryan L, Chen Z, et al. Phthalate exposure and human semen parameters. *Epidemiology.* 2003;14(3):269-277.

Environmental News Service. *Mercury Emissions Up at Coal Burning Power Plants.* November 21, 2008. www.ens-newswire.com/ens/nov2008/2008-11-21-092.asp (Accessed April 4, 2010).

Environmental Working Group. *Body Burden: the Pollution in Newborns.* July 14, 2005. Washington, DC. http://www.ewg.org/reports/bodyburden2/

Environmental Working Group. The Campaign for Safe Cosmetics. May 12, 2010. *Not so Sexy; The Health Risks of Secret Chemicals in Fragrance.* www.SafeCosmetics.org.

Environmental Working Group. *Chemical Families; Haloacetic acids.* www.ewg.org/chemindex/term/513. (Accessed April 6, 2010).

Environmental Working Group. *Not So Sexy; Hidden Chemicals in Perfume and Cologne.* www.ewg.org/notsosexy?utm_source=fragrance&utm_medium=email&utm_content=first-link&utm_campaign=toxic. (Accessed May 15, 2010).

Environmental Working Group. Over *300 Pollutants in U.S. Tap Water.* www.ewg.org/tapwater/home. (Accessed April 6, 2010).

Environmental Working Group. *Shopper's Guide to Pesticides.* www.foodnews.org.

Environmental Working Group. Skin Deep Cosmetic Safety Database. www.cosmeticsdatabase.com/special/.../ingredients.php. (Accessed April 15, 2010).

Environmental Working Group, HCWH (Health Care without Harm), WVE (Women's Voices for the Earth) (Houlihan, Brody, Schwan). *Not Too Pretty: Phthalates, beauty products, and the FDA.* July 10, 2002. Washington, DC. http://www.ewg.org/reports/nottoopretty/

Farlow CH. *Dying to Look Good; The Disturbing Truth About What's Really in Your Cosmetics, Toiletries, and Personal Care Products...And What You Can Do About It.* Escondido, CA: KISS For Health Publishing, 2006.

Fitzgerald R. *The Hundred-Year Lie; How to Protect Yourself From the Chemicals That Are Destroying Your Health.* New York, NY: Plume, 2007.

Food and Drug Administration (FDA). 2000. *Clearing Up Cosmetic Confusion.* FDA Consumer, May - June 1998. Revised May 1998 and August 2000. http://www.cfsan.fda.gov/~dms/fdconfus.html

Freese W, and Schubert D. Safety testing and regulation of genetically engineered foods. *Biotechnology and Genetic Engineering Reviews.* Nov 2004;21.

Fromme H, Tittlemier SA, Volkel W, Wilhelm M, and Twardella D. Perfluorinated compounds—exposure assessment for the general population in Western countries. *Int J Hyg Environ Health.* 2009;212(3):239–270.

GMO Compass. *Dairy Products and Eggs.* www.gmo-compass.org/.../29.dairy_products_eggs_genetic_engineering.html. (Accessed March 10, 2010).

Hainer R. *Study Links BPA in Plastics to Erectile Dysfunction.* November 11, 2009. www.cnn.com/health. (Accessed April 6, 2010).

Hanson KM, Gratton E, and Bardeen CJ. Sunscreen enhancement of UV-induced reactive oxygen species in the skin. *Free radical biology & medicine.* 2006;41(8):1205-1212.

Hayden C, Roberts M, and Benson H. Systemic absorption of sunscreen after topical application. *Lancet.* 1997;350(Sep):863-864.

Hayden CGJ, Cross SE, Anderson C, Saunders NA, and Roberts MS. Sunscreen penetration of human skin and related keratinocyte toxicity after topical application. *Skin pharmacology and physiology.* 2005;18(4):170-174.

Heindel JJ, vom Saal FS. Role of nutrition and environmental endocrine disrupting chemicals during the perinatal period on the aetiology of obesity. *Mol Cell Endocrinol.* 2009;304(1-2):90-96.

Hill AB. *The environment and disease: association or causation?* Proceeding of the Royal Society of Medicine 1965;58:295-300.

Hotchkiss AK, Rider CV, Blystone CR, Wilson VS, Hartig PC, Ankley GT, Foster PM, Gray CL, and Gray LE. Fifteen years after "Wingspread" – environmental endocrine disrupters and human and wildlife health: where we are today and where we need to go. *Toxicol Sci.* 2008;105(2):235-259.

Interior Landscape Plants for Indoor Air Pollution Abatement. National Aeronautics and Space Administration study. September 15, 1989.

Jansson T, and Loden M. Strategy to decrease the risk of adverse effects of fragrance ingredients in cosmetic products. *American journal of contact dermatitis.* 2001;12(3):166-169.

Johnson E, and Lucey, A. "Major Technological Advances and Trends in Cheese." *J. Dairy Sci.* 2006;89(4):1174–1178.

Jugan ML, Levi Y, and Blondeau JP. Endocrine disruptors and thyroid hormone physiology. *Biochem Pharmacol.* 2010;79(7):939-947.

Kamrin M. *Traces of Environmental Chemicals in the Human Body: Are They a Risk to Health? 2003.* New York: American Council on Science and Health. Available: http://www.acsh.org/publications/pubID.195/pub_detail.asp. (Accessed March 3, 2010).

Katelaris CH, and Peake JE. Allergy and the skin: eczema and chronic urticaria. *The Medical journal of Australia.* 2006;185(9):517-522.

Kilic A, and Aday M. A three generational study with genetically modified Bt corn in rats: biochemical and histopathological investigation. *Food Chem. Toxicol.* 2008;46(3):1164-1170.

"Lake Roosevelt toxins could become airborne." Associated Press. August 23, 2004.

Lofstedt R. *The precautionary principle: risk, regulation and politics.* Merton College: Oxford, 2002.

Main KM, Mortensen GK, Kaleva MM, Boisen KA, Damgaard IN, Chellakooty M, et al. Human breast milk contamination with phthalates and alterations of endogenous reproductive hormones in infants three months of age. *Environmental health perspectives*. 2006;114(2):270-276.

Malatesta M, Boraldi F, Annovi G, et al. A long-term study on female mice fed on a genetically modified soybean: effects on liver ageing. *Histochem Cell Biol*. 2008;130:967-977.

Malkan S. *Not Just a Pretty Face*. Gabriola Island, Canada: New Society Publishers, 2007.

Mayeda J. "Contaminated Arctic Only Looks Pristine." *San Francisco Chronicle*. May 22, 2005.

McClure R, and Paulson T. "Toxins fill our air, study finds". *Seattle Post*. 20 April 2002. D3.

Millqvist E, and Lowhagen O. Placebo-controlled challenges with perfume in patients with asthma-like symptoms. *Allergy*. 1996;51(6):434-439.

Nagel JE, Fuscaldo JT, and Fireman P. Paraben allergy. *JAMA*. 1977;237(15):1594-1595.

Naidenko O, et al. Bottle Water Contains Disinfection Byproducts, Fertilizer Residue, and Pain Medication. Environmental Working Group. October 2008. www.ewg.org/reports/bottledwater. (Accessed April 6, 2010).

Nakazawa DJ. *The Autoimmune Epidemic*. New York, NY: Touchstone, 2008.

National Academy of Sciences. *"Pesticides in the Diets of Infants and Children."* National Academy Press, 1993.

National Cancer Institute, Division of Extramural Activities, President's Cancer Panel. 2008-2009 Annual Report, April 2010. *Reducing Environmental Cancer Risk, What We Can Do Now*. pcp.cancer.gov. (Accessed May 2, 2010).

National Center for Health Statistics (NCHS). National Health and Nutrition Examination Survey: Lab Methods 2005–2006. http://www.cdc.gov/nchs/data/nhanes/nhanes_05_06/pfc_d_met.pdf. (Accessed December 4, 2009).

National Institute of Health, The autoimmune disease Coordinating Committee, Report to Congress. *Progress in Autoimmune Diseases Research*. March 2005. www.niaid.nih.gov/topics/autoimmune/Documents/adccfinal.pdf. (Accessed April 15, 2010).

Netherwood T, et al. "Assessing the survival of transgenic planic plant DNA in the human gastrointestinal tract." *Nature Biotechnology* 22 (2004):2.

Oliveria SA, Saraiya M, Geller AC, Heneghan MK, and Jorgensen C. Sun exposure and risk of melanoma. *Archives of disease in childhood*. 2006;91(2):131-138.

Pazzaglia M, and Tosti A. Allergic contact dermatitis from 3-iodo-2-propynyl-butylcarbamate in a cosmetic cream. *Contact dermatitis*. 1999;41(5):290.

Pont AR, Charron AR, and Brand RM. Active ingredients in sunscreens act as topical penetration enhancers for the herbicide 2,4-dichlorophenoxyacetic acid. *Toxicology and applied pharmacology.* 2004;195(3):348-354.

Prins GS. Endocrine disruptors and prostate cancer risk. *Endocr Relat Cancer.* 2008;15(3):649-656.

Public Employees for Environmental Responsibility (PEER). "Genetic Genie: The Premature Commercial Release of Genetically Engineered Bacteria." September 1995.

Rastogi SC, Johansen JD, and Menne T. Natural ingredients based cosmetics. Content of selected fragrance sensitizers. *Contact Dermatitis.* 1996;34(6):423-426.

Rissler J, and Mellon M. *The Ecological Risks of Engineered Crops.* Cambridge: MIT Press, 1996.

Routledge EJ, Parker J, Odum J, Ashby J, and Sumpter JP. Some alkyl hydroxy benzoate preservatives (parabens) are estrogenic. *Toxicology and applied pharmacology.* 1998;153(1):12-19.

Rüdel H, Böhmer W, and Schröter-Kermani C. Retrospective monitoring of synthetic musk compounds in aquatic biota from German rivers and coastal areas. *J. Environ. Monit.* 2006;8(8):812-823.

Scheinman PL. Exposing covert fragrance chemicals. *Am J Contact Dermat.* 2001;12(4):225-228.

Scheinman PL. The foul side of fragrance-free products. *J Am Acad Dermatol.* 2000;42(6):1087.

Scheinman PL. Prevalence of fragrance allergy. *Dermatology.* 2002;205(1):98-102.

Schlumpf M, Cotton B, Conscience M, Haller V, Steinmann B, and Lichtensteiger W. In vitro and in vivo estrogenicity of UV screens. *Environmental health perspectives.* 2001;109(3):239-244.

Schlumpf M, Schmid P, Durrer S, Conscience M, Maerkel K, Henseler M, et al. Endocrine activity and developmental toxicity of cosmetic UV filters--an update. *Toxicology.* 2004;205(1-2):113-122.

Scientific Committee On Cosmetic Products And Non-Food Products (SCCPNFP). 2000. An Initial List Of Perfumery Materials Which Must Not Form Part Of Fragrances Compounds Used In Cosmetic Products. SCCNFP/0320/00, final May 2000.

Sexton K, Needham L, and Pirkle J. Human biomonitoring of environmental chemicals: measuring chemicals in human tissues is the "gold standard" for assessing exposure to pollution. *Am Sci.* 2004;92:38–42..

Smith JM. *Genetic Roulette; The Documented Health Risks of Genetically Engineered Foods.* Fairfield, Iowa: Yes! Books, 2007.

Society of Toxicology. The safety of genetically modified foods produced through biotechnology. *Toxicol. Sci.* 2003;71:2-8.

Soni MG, Burdock GA, Taylor SL, and Greenberg NA. Safety assessment of propyl paraben: a review of the published literature. *Food chemistry and toxicology.* 2001;39(6):513-532.

Steingraber S. *The Falling Age of Puberty: What we know, what we need to know.* Breast Cancer Fund. August 2007. http://www.breastcancerfund.org/site/pp.asp?c=kwKXLdPaE&b=3266509. (Accessed January 26, 2010).

Stokstad E. Pollution gets personal. *Science.* 2004;304:1892–1894.

Swan SH, Main KM, Liu F, Stewart SL, Kruse RL, Calafat AM, et al. Decrease in anogenital distance among male infants with prenatal phthalate exposure. *Environmental health perspectives.* 2005;113(8):1056-1061.

Tennessee Valley Authority. *On the Air; Mercury Emissions.* www.tva.gov/environment/air/ontheair/merc_emis.htm. (Accessed April 5, 2010).

Thornton JW, McCally M, and Houlihan J. Biomonitoring of industrial pollutants: health and policy implications of the chemical body burden. *Public health reports.* 2002;117(4):315-323.

Townsend M. "Why Soya is a Hidden Destroyer." *Daily Express.* 12 March 1999.

2005 Dietary Guidelines for Americans. Center for Nutrition Policy and Promotion, U.S. Department of Agriculture.

Understanding the Role of Science in Regulation. The Wingspread Statement and the European Union. *Environmental Health Perspectives.* 2009 Mar;Volume 117 Number 3.

U.S. Department of Health and Human Services and U. S. Environmental Protection Agency, FDA/Center for Food Safety & Applied Nutrition. *What You Need to Know About Mercury in Fish and Shellfish.* March 2004.

U.S. Environmental Protection Agency. Puget Sound Clean Air Agency Solutions-Case Study. www.epa.gov/p2/pubs/casestudies/pugetsound.htm. (Accessed March 5, 2010).

U.S. Environmental Protection Agency. Summary of Toxic Substances Control Act, 15 U.S.C. 2601 et seq. (1976). www.epa.gov/lawsregs/laws/tsca. (Accessed March 24, 2010).

Vidal J. *GM Genes Found in Human Gut. The Guardian.* July 17, 2002. http://www.guardian.co.uk/gmdebate/Story/0,2763,756666,00.html. (Accessed April 7, 2010).

Williams F. Toxic breast milk? *New York Times Magazine.* 2005. http://www.nytimes.com/2005/01/09/magazine/09TOXIC.htm. (Accessed March 2, 2010).

Wolff MS, Teitelbaum SL, Windham G, Pinney SM, Britton JA, Chelimo C, et al. Pilot study of urinary biomarkers of phytoestrogens, phthalates, and phenols in girls. *Environmental health perspectives.* 2007;115(1):116-121.

World Health Organization. Total Diet Studies: A Recipe for Safer Food. 2005. Geneva: World Health Organization. http://www.who.int/foodsafety/chem/TDS_recipe_2005_en.pdf. (Accessed March 9, 2010).

Chapter 9 References

Abou-Donia MB, El-Masry EM, Abdel-Rahman AA, McLendon RE, and Schiffman SS. Splenda alters gut microflora and increases intestinal p-glycoprotein and cytochrome p-450 in male rats. *J Toxicol Environ Health A.* 2008;71(21):1415-1429.

Alafuzoff I, et al. "Blood-Brain Barrier in Alzheimer Dementia and in Non-Demented Elderly. An Immunocytochemical Study." *Acta Neuropathologica.* 1987. Volume 73, No. 2:160-166.

Atlas N. *The Vegetarian 5-Ingredient Gourmet,* 200 Simple Recipes and Dozens of Healthy Menus for Eating Well Every Day. New York, NY: Broadway Books, 2001.

Bellero L. March 25, 2010. *A sweet problem: Princeton researchers find that high-fructose corn syrup prompts considerably more weight gain.* http://www.princeton.edu/main/news/archive/S26/91/22K07/index.xml?section=topstories. (Accessed April 19, 2010).

The BioInitiative Working Group Report. August 31, 2007. *BioInitiative Report: A Rationale for a Biologically-based Public Exposure Standard for Electromagnetic Fields (ELF and R).* www.bioinitiative.org/report/index.htm. (Accessed April 12, 2010).

Blank M. "Preface." *Pathophysiology* 2009 16(2–3):67–69.

Blaylock RI. *Excitotoxins: The Taste That Kills.* Santa Fe, NM: Health Press, 1997.

Blum A, Front E, and Peleg A. Periodontal care may improve systemic inflammation. *Clin Invest Med.* 2007;30(3):E114-117.

Blundell JE, and Hill AJ. "Paradoxical effects of an intense sweetener (aspartame) on appetite." *The Lancet.* 1986 Volume 1:1092-1093.

Boehm TK, and Scannapieco FA. The epidemiology, consequences and management of periodontal disease in older adults. *J Am Dent Assoc.* 2007 Sep;138 (Suppl):26S-33S.

Boor PJ, et al. "Methylamine Metabolism to Formaldehyde by Vascular Semicarbazide-Sensitive Amine Oxidase." *Toxicology.* 1992 Volume 73;No. 3:251-258.

Brand RM, Pike J, Wilson RM, and Charron AR. Sunscreens containing physical UV blockers can increase transdermal absorption of pesticides. *Toxicol Ind Health.* 2003 Feb;19(1):9-16.

Brand RM, Spalding M, and Mueller C. Sunscreens can increase dermal penetration of 2,4-dichlorophenoxyacetic acid. *J Toxicol Clin Toxicol.* 2002;40(7):827-832.

Brody JE. *"Sweetener Worries Some Scientists."* Science Times. February 5, 1985. Reprinted in Congressional Record (1985a: S5493-S5494).

Cabrera C, Artacho R, and Gimenez R. Beneficial effects of green tea—a review. *J Am Coll Nutr.* 2006 Apr;25(2):79-99.

Calafat AM, Ye X, Wong LY, Reidy JA, and Needham LL. Exposure of the U.S. population to bisphenol A and 4-tertiary-octylphenol: 2003-2004. *Environ Health Perspect.* 2008 Jan;116(1):39-44.

Cannell J. *Vitamin D Newletter.* August 2006.

Carper J. *Food: Your Miracle Medicine, How Food Can Prevent and Cure Over 100 Symptoms and Problems.* New York, NY: Harper Paperbacks, 1993.

Dowd J. *The Vitamin D Cure.* Hoboken, New Jersey: John Wiley & Sons, Inc., 2008.

Draelos ZD. Are sunscreens safe? *J Cosmet Dermatol.* 2010 Mar;9(1):1-2.

Environmental Working Group. *EWG's 2010 Sunscreen Guide.* www.ewg. org/2010sunscreen/?inlist=Y&utm_source=sunscreenresend&utm_medium=email&utm_. (Accessed May 28, 2010).

Environmental Working Group. *Nanomaterials and Hormone Disruptors in Sunscreens.* www.ewg. org/2010sunscreen/full-report/nanomaterials-and-hormone-disruptors-in-sunscreens/. (Accessed May 28, 2010).

Environmental Working Group. *Not So Sexy; Hidden Chemicals in Perfume and Cologne.* www. ewg. org/notsosexy (Accessed May 14, 2010).

Food and Drug Administration (FDA). "Generally Recognized as Safe (GRAS)." http://www. fda.gov/Food/FoodIngredientsPackaging/GenerallyRecognizedasSafeGRAS/default.htm (Accessed April 14, 2010).

Genco R, Offenbacher S, and Beck J. Periodontal disease and cardiovascular disease. Epidemiology and possible mechanisms. *J Am Dent Assoc.* 2002 Jun;133:14S-22S.

Genco RJ, Grossi SG, Ho A, Nishimura F, Murayama Y. A proposed model linking inflammation to obesity, diabetes, and periodontal infections. *J Periodontol.* 2005 Nov;76(11 Suppl):2075-2084.

Grossi S. Smoking and stress: common denominators for periodontal disease, heart disease, and diabetes mellitus. *Compend Contin Educ Dent Suppl.* 2000;(30):31-39.

Grossi S. Treatment of periodontal disease and control of diabetes: an assessment of the evidence and need for future research. *Ann Periodontol.* 2001 Dec;6(1):138-145.

Grossi S, and Genco R. Periodontal disease and diabetes mellitus: a two way relationship. *Ann Periodontol.* 1998 Jul;3(1):51-61.

Haas EM. *The Staying Healthy Shoppers Guide; Feed Your Family Safely by Learning to Avoid: Additives, Preservatives, Pesticides, Pathogens, Processed Foods, and More...* Berkeley, CA: Celestial Arts, 1999.

Hahn RA. The nocebo phenomenon: concept, evidence, and implications for public health. *Prev Med.* 1997 Sep-Oct;26(5 Pt 1):607-611.

Hamer M, Witte DR, Mosdøl A, Marmot MG, and Brunner EJ. Prospective study of coffee and tea consumption in relation to risk of type 2 diabetes mellitus among men and women: the Whitehall II study. *Br J Nutr.* 2008 Nov;100(5):1046-1053.

Haraszthy V, Zambon J, Trevisan M, Zeid M, and Genco R. Identification of periodontal pathogens in atheromatous plaques. *J Periodontol.* 2000 Oct;71(10):1554-1060.

Huxley R, Lee CM, Barzi F, Timmermeister L, Czernichow S, Perkovic V, Grobbee DE, Batty D, and Woodward M. Coffee, decaffeinated coffee, and tea consumption in relation to incident type 2 diabetes mellitus: a systematic review with meta-analysis. *Arch Intern Med.* 2009 Dec 14;169(22):2053-2063.

Janjua NR, Kongshoj B, Andersson AM, and Wulf HC. Sunscreens in human plasma and urine after repeated whole-body topical application. *J Eur Acad Dermatol Venereol.* 2008 Apr;22(4):456-461.

Jeffcoat M, Lewis C, Reddy M, Wang CY, and Redford M. Post-menopausal bone loss and its relationship to oral bone loss. *Periodontol.* 2000;23:94-102.

Krall E, Dawson-Hughes B, Papas A, and Garcia R. Tooth loss and skeletal bone density in healthy postmenopausal women. *Osteoporosis Int.* 1994 Mar;4(2):104-109.

Krejci C, and Bissada N. Women's health issues and their relationship to periodontitis. *J Am Dent Assoc.* 2002 Mar;133(3):323-329.

Lappe JM, Travers-Gustafson D, Davies KM, et al. Vitamin D and calcium supplementation reduces cancer risk: results of a randomized trial. *Am J Clin Nutr.* 2007; 85(6):1586-1591.

Lee J, O'Keefe JH, Bell D, Hensrud DD, and Holick MF. "Vitamin D Deficiency: An Important, Common, and Easily Treatable Cardiovascular Risk Factor?" *Journal of American College of Cardiology.* 2008;Vol. 52, No. 24.

Looker AC, Dawson-Hughes B, Calvo MS, Gunter EW, and Sahyoun NR. Serum 25-hydroxyvitamin D status of adolescents and adults in two seasonal subpopulations from NHANES III. *Bone* 2002;30:771-777.

Loos BG, Craandijk J, Hoek FJ, Wertheim-van Dillen PM, and van der Velden U. Elevation of systemic markers related to cardiovascular disease in peripheral blood of periodontitis patients. *J Periodontol.* 2000 Oct;71(10):1528-1534.

Lynch H, and Milgrom P. Xylitol and dental caries: an overview for clinicians. *J Calif Dent Assoc.* 2003 Mar;31(3):205-209.

Machado M, Koch AJ, Willardson JM, dos Santos FC, Curty VM, and Pereira LN. Caffeine does not augment markers of muscle damage or leukocytosis following resistance exercise. *Int J Sports Physiol Perform.* 2010 Mar;5(1):18-26.

Merchant A, Pitiphant W, Rimm E, and Joshipura K. Increased physical activity decreases periodontitis risk in men. *Eur J Epidemiol.* 2003;18(9):891-898.

Mercola J, and Herman J. *Dark Deception; Discover the Truth About the Benefits of Sunlight Exposure.* Hoffman Estates, IL; Mercola.com, 2008.

Michaud DS, Joshipura K, Giovannucci E, Fuchs CS. A prospective study of periodontal disease and pancreatic cancer in US male health professionals. *J Natl Cancer Inst.* 2007 Jan 17;99(2):171-175.

Michaud DS, Liu Y, Meyer M, Giovannucci E, and Joshipura K. Periodontal disease, tooth loss, and cancer risk in male health professionals: a prospective cohort study. *Lancet Oncol.* 2008 Jun;9(6):550-558.

Monte WC. "Aspartame: Methanol and the Public Health." *Journal of Applied Nutrition.* 1984;36(1):42-53.

Mustapha IZ, Debrey S, Oladubu M, and Ugarte R. Markers of systemic bacterial exposure in periodontal disease and cardiovascular disease risk: a systematic review and meta-analysis. *J Periodontol.* 2007 Dec;78(12):2289-2302.

Pack AR. Folate mouthwash: effects on established gingivitis in periodontal patients. *J Clin Periodontol.* 1984 Oct;11(9):619-628.

Pischon N, Heng N, Bernimoulin JP, et al. Obesity, inflammation, and periodontal disease. *J Dent Res.* 2007 May;86(5):400-409.

Pont AR, Charron AR, and Brand RM. Active ingredients in sunscreens act as topical penetration enhancers for the herbicide 2,4-dichlorophenoxyacetic acid. *Toxicology and applied pharmacology.* 2004;195(3):348-354.

Ridker P, Rifai N, Rose L, Buring J, and Cook N. Comparison of C-reactive protein and low-density lipoprotein cholesterol levels in the prediction of first cardiovascular events. *N Engl J Med.* 2002 Nov 14;347(20):1557-1565.

Scannapieco F, and Ho A. Potential associations between chronic respiratory disease and periodontal disease: Analysis of National Health and Nutrition Examination Survey III. *J Periodontol.* 2001 Jan;72(1):50-56.

Sies H, and Stahl W. Nutritional protection against skin damage from sunlight. *Annu Rev Nutr.* 2004;24:173-200.

Sleiman M, Gundel LA, Pankow JF, Jacob P 3rd, Singer BC, and Destaillats H. Formation of carcinogens indoors by surface-mediated reactions of nicotine with nitrous acid, leading to potential thirdhand smoke hazards. *Proc Natl Acad Sci U S A.* 2010 Apr 13,107(15):6576-6581.

Tolleson WH, Cherng SH, Xia Q, Boudreau M, Yin JJ, Wamer WG, Howard PC, Yu H, and Fu PP. Photodecomposition and phototoxicity of natural retinoids. *Int J Environ Res Public Health.* 2005 Apr;2(1):147-155.

Vasconcelos LC, Sampaio FC, Sampaio MC, et al. Minimum inhibitory concentration of adherence of Punica granatum Linn (pomegranate) gel against S. mutans, S. mitis and C. albicans. *Braz Dent J.* 2006;17(3):223-227.

Wilkinson EG, Arnold RM, and Folkers K. Bioenergetics in clinical medicine. VI. adjunctive treatment of periodontal disease with coenzyme Q10. *Res Commun Chem Pathol Pharmacol.* 1976 Aug;14(4):715-719.

Williams RC, Barnett AH, Claffey N, et al. The potential impact of periodontal disease on general health: a consensus view. *Curr Med Res Opin.* 2008 Apr 30.

Wood N, and Johnson R. Recovery of Periopathogenic Bacteria From Embalmed Human Cadavers. *Clinical Anatomy In Press.*

Wurtman RJ, and Ritter-Walker E. *"Dietary Phenylalanine and Brain Function."* Proceedings of the First International Meeting on Dietary Phenylalanine and Brain Function. Washington, DC. May 8, 1987.

Chapter 10 References

Buettner D. *The Blue Zones; Lessons for Living Longer From the People Who've Lived the Longest.* Washington, DC: National Geographic, 2008.

Kurzweil R. *The Singularity is Near; When Humans Transcend Biology.* New York, NY: Penguin Books, 2005.

Kurzweil R, and Grossman T. *Fantastic Voyage; Live Long Enough To Live Forever.* New York, NY: Penguin Books, 2004.

RECOMMENDED

RESOURCES

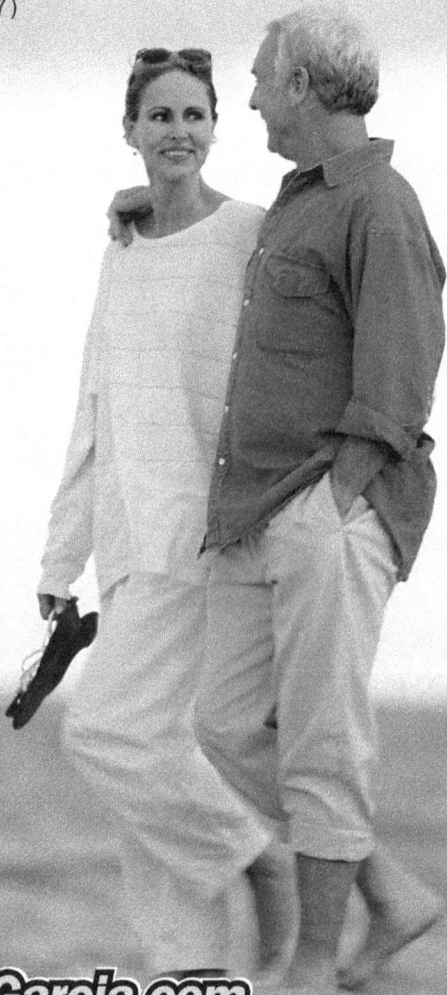

body ⊗ logic md ®

1200 POLARIS PARKWAY, SUITE 100

COLUMBUS, OHIO 43240

1-877-501-4**ATP** (4287)

MANAGERS:

MICHELE ALBANS

TRACEY HOLCOMB

www.DrRogerGarcia.com

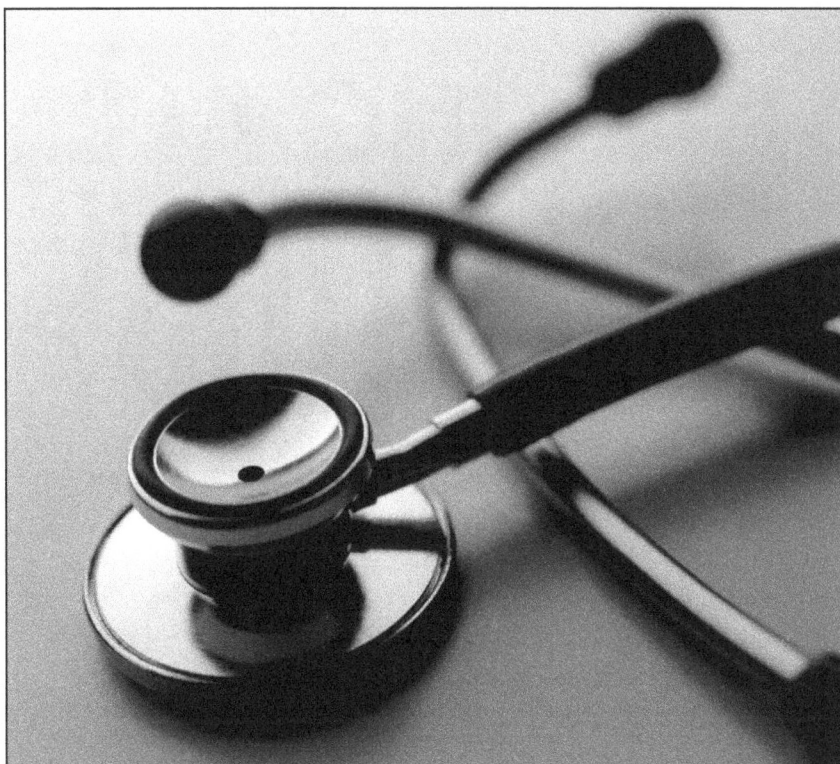

POLARIS | *URGENT CARE*

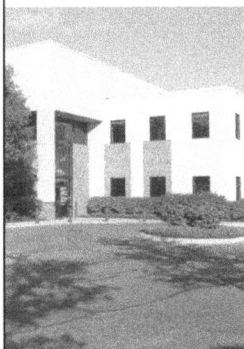

1120 POLARIS PARKWAY

COLUMBUS, OHIO 43240

PHONE: 614-847-1120

FAX: 614-847-1205

MANAGERS:

LEE MAYLE

JOE ANNIN

www.polarisurgentcare.com

OPEN 7 DAYS A WEEK (9 AM TO 9PM)

BELLEVUE
HOSPITAL

1400 WEST MAIN ST.

BELLEVUE, OHIO 44811

(419) 484-4040

BELLEVUEHOSPITAL.COM

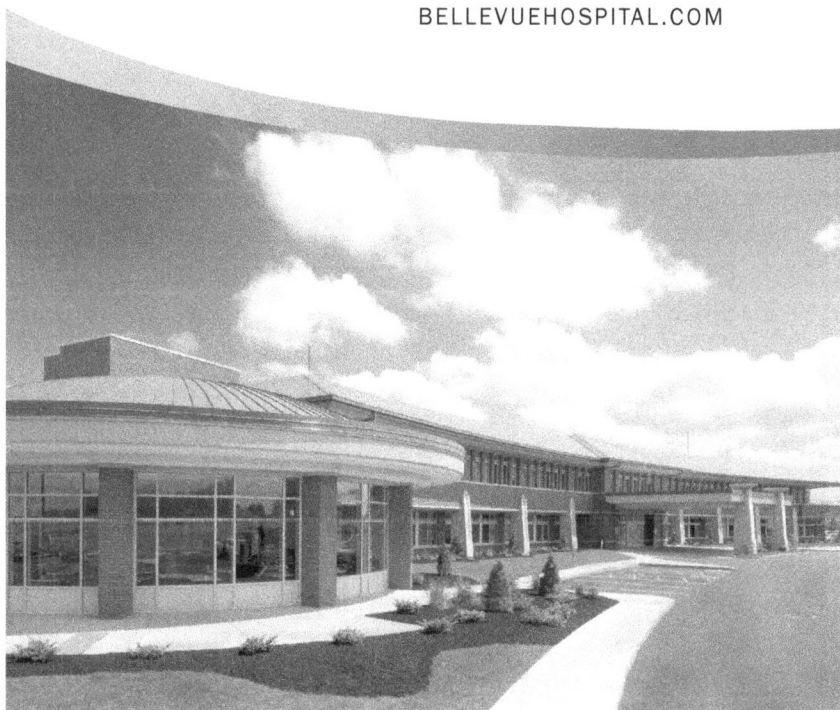

NORTH CENTRAL EMS

12513 US ROUTE 250 NORTH
MILAN, OHIO 44846
1-800-589-2515

NORTHCENTRALEMS.COM

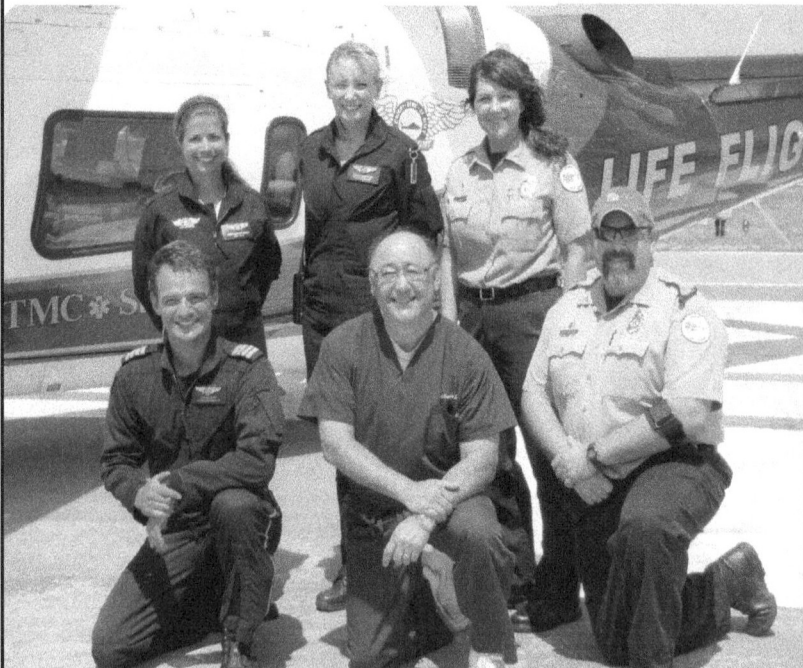

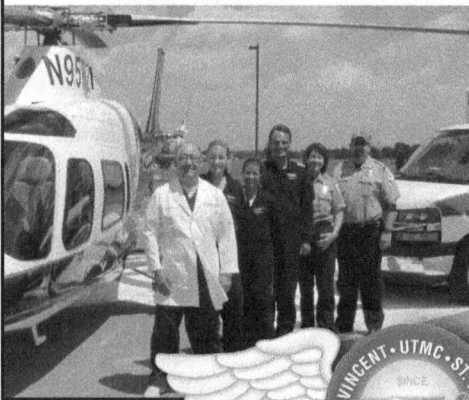

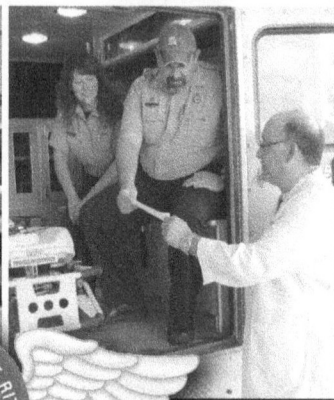

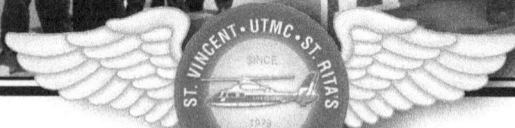

ST. VINCENT • UTMC • ST. RITA'S
SINCE
1979

LIFE FLIGHT

www.ingramcontent.com/pod-product-compliance
Lightning Source LLC
Chambersburg PA
CBHW051726260326
41914CB00031B/1755/J